STRONG

Thorsons
An imprint of HarperCollins*Publishers*
1 London Bridge Street
London SE1 9GF
www.harpercollins.co.uk

HarperCollins*Publishers*
Macken House, 39/40 Mayor Street Upper
Dublin 1, D01 C9W8, Ireland

First published by Thorsons 2025

1 3 5 7 9 10 8 6 4 2

A catalogue record of this book is available from the British Library
ISBN 978-0-00-870136-9

Printed and bound in the UK using 100% renewable electricity at CPI Group (UK) Ltd

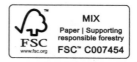

STRONG

The Definitive Guide to Active Ageing

JACQUELINE HOOTON

Thorsons

In loving memory of my brother Jonathan, and those who departed too young, too soon and will never grow older with us.

CONTENTS

PREFACE

'Don't get old, dear,' my grandmother used to say to me. Yet she enjoyed reasonably good health in her later years, lived independently, and was fully mobile until her death in 1998 at 88 years old. I was very close to my grandmother; our birthdays just one day apart – hers on 10 February and mine on 11 February. As a little girl, she used to tell me, 'When you grow up, we'll go out and paint the town red and have a joint birthday celebration.' Sadly, we never got to do that. Instead, I took a call from my mother on my thirty-fifth birthday, on 11 February 1998, to tell me my grandmother had passed away in the night. We will never know her exact time of death, but I prefer to imagine she died before midnight, on her own birthday, with amazing synchronicity.

Perhaps you have heard a similar lament from older adults, maybe you've even thought this or said it yourself. Growing older is often something that is feared. We are bombarded with negative images and ideas about older people, and as a result we often believe that deterioration is inevitable and our lives will become harder and less enjoyable with each passing year.

I didn't get to 'paint the town red' with my grandmother, but every year on my birthday I go to the gym and enjoy a workout. This habit acknowledges the important impact that exercise and physical activity has on my health and sets my intention for the year ahead. And if my grandmother was alive today I'd tell her, 'I'm growing older and it's okay!'

There's another, poignant reason why I'm grateful to be growing older.

In 1984, my eighteen-year-old brother Jonathan died whilst on active service with the Royal Navy. He was on a tour of duty in the

Falkland Islands following the Falklands War. A missile misfired and he was caught in the efflux. Jonathan sustained 60 per cent burns and died in hospital three days later, on 1 February, a few hours before the military aircraft on which my parents were being transported touched down in Port Stanley.

Jonathan's death, just before my twenty-first birthday, had a profound effect on me. The grief of losing my younger brother was unimaginably painful, the manner of his death the stuff of nightmares. The impact on my parents was understandably traumatic. For a long time, I thought their grief would kill them and rob me of them too.

The death of a young person, especially someone we love, can significantly influence our thoughts about life. It's a privilege to get old. The older I get, the more this resonates. I don't take life for granted, I know things can change in a heartbeat and, far from fearing growing older, I am determined to embrace each year and appreciate all the years I get to live. The years my brother was denied.

MY FITNESS JOURNEY

Working as an antenatal teacher for the National Childbirth Trust (NCT) in the early 1990s was the spark that ignited my interest in female health and wellbeing, and studying to become a fitness instructor was the next logical step for me. I'm a personal trainer with a career that spans over two decades, in which I've focused on empowering women to make informed decisions about their health and fitness.

Growing up I enjoyed gymnastics, ballet, roller skating, hockey and riding my bike everywhere. But physical education (PE) at secondary school was torturous for me, as it was for many of my peers.

It was the 1970s; the school had shared communal showers and soulless concrete-block changing rooms. Lycra, invented in 1958, had yet to make it into sportswear for girls; our PE kit consisted of a shapeless and scratchy Aertex shirt, a wraparound pleated sports skirt (which easily came undone) and thick, navy-blue knickers to wear over our regular underwear (on account of the unreliability of our wraparound skirts!).

It was rounders and athletics in the summer, cross-country, hockey and netball in the winter. And perhaps we'd have felt better about these activities if it hadn't included the stress of team selection. The teacher always selected the same two girls she deemed sufficiently sporty and 'good' at PE as team captains. The rest of the class would wait anxiously while the 'sporty' girls took turns picking their preferred team members.

My experience of school PE is far from unique – many of the women I have worked with over the years have shared their own loathing of PE with me. An early negative association with physical activity and sport can set the course for an ongoing fear and dread of exercise. In recent years I have reconnected with old school friends, and one of them was completely astounded to hear about my work now as a personal trainer and my passion for fitness and exercise, correctly remembering my disdain for PE. It was nothing to do with loathing physical activity, exercise and moving my body, it was down to the ugly and uncomfortable sports kit, coupled with a fear of humiliation and shame.

In the early 1980s, sexism and misogyny were rife in society and the workplace – we were living #MeToo daily. I had just finished a euphemistically-named 'fun run' for a work-related event, where male members of staff patronised me by saying I'd never run far in heels. This pushed me to try to prove that I was capable of running, albeit not in heels! It would take another 30 years for me to realise there are better ways of 'showing them' than running in an event I'd had no training for. Predictably, things didn't go quite the way I had hoped during the fun run. As I half-ran, half-stumbled over the finish line I was greeted by jeers from the male members of staff. I swore I'd never run again.

But I was wrong; not only would I run again, I'd take part in many more running events, including one of the most iconic races in the world – the London Marathon.

In 1989, at 26 years old, I gave birth to my first baby, a son we named Tobias. I looked at him in his car seat on my arrival home from hospital with my husband Chris, and the terrifying realisation that I was responsible for another human life dawned on me. I knew I had to look after myself to take care of my baby, even though I wasn't too sure what that entailed. So, when I saw *Jane Fonda's Original Workout* video in Woolworths, I decided this might be a good place to start. With social media yet to be invented, no YouTube or Instagram, Jane Fonda is now widely recognised as a trailblazer for workout videos, DVDs and home exercise.

For the first time in my life, I started to enjoy exercise as I followed Jane Fonda's routines. I found the workouts made me feel energised and lifted my mood. I felt 'fitter' and began to find the workouts easier.

I had a newfound respect for my body. It made me reflect on my experience of childbirth and the NCT classes I'd attended beforehand. So, I decided to train to become an NCT antenatal teacher, to enable new mums to make informed choices, understand the physical changes that are happening to their bodies and prepare for the birth of their babies.

In 1992, when my son was three years old, we moved with my husband's work from Eastcote in Hillingdon to Marlborough in Wiltshire. Our house was at the top of a steepish hill. Marlborough Leisure Centre was nestled at the bottom of the hill, and it quickly became a favourite venue for toddler activities and swimming with my son, as well as exercise classes for me. Twice weekly I attended the centre's ladies' mornings. The two-hour session included an aerobics class and was followed by a choice of activities, including badminton, trampolining and the use of a very small gym.

In June 1994 I gave birth at home to my second baby – my daughter, Poppy. Education and information about postnatal recovery was limited in the early 1990s. Postnatal exercise classes didn't exist in the way they do today, and the fitness industry didn't cater for specific female health issues, like pregnancy and menopause. So my fitness routine in the early weeks following Poppy's delivery was walking up and down the hill we lived on, taking my son to school.

By 1995 we were on the move again and we headed to Chalfont-St-Giles, in Buckinghamshire. Yet again we lived at the top of a very steep hill, and I would do the round trip walking to and from school for drop off and collection twice daily, with Poppy in the pushchair and Tobias walking. I didn't know it at the time, but walking up a steep incline while pushing the weight of a growing toddler, and accumulating 5 miles and over an hour of walking every day is a great way to build stamina and support cardiovascular health! But when a new gym opened in the area, with a creche, I knew it was the perfect opportunity to add some structured exercise to my life.

Although not of the standard of gyms nowadays, and with no free weights, the range of resistance machines on offer meant I got my first taste of training to improve strength. My gym induction at the time hadn't included how to use the treadmill, but I can remember looking at the treadmills and the other gym users running on them and being curious. So I decided to figure out how to use one a few weeks later, and a cautious walk turned into a gentle jog, then a brief run. The embarrassment of my failed fun run at 18 a distant memory, now I was simply running for my own sense of achievement and enjoyment.

When I became pregnant again in 1997, aged 34, with my third child, I was the fittest I'd ever been on account of the daily walking to and from school, regular gym sessions and the line dancing classes I'd recently joined. My son Gabriel was born at home in the October.

With Tobias in school and Poppy attending nursery, I was able to return to the gym for a couple of mornings a week whilst Gabriel was looked after in the creche. I was thoroughly exhausted though; Gabriel had a reflux issue that made him a very uncomfortable baby who had trouble sleeping. Exercise during this period became more about supporting my mental wellbeing and managing the stress of sleepless nights than fitness. Then, when Gabriel was just four months old, my beloved grandmother died. It was the day after her funeral when we discovered a new house being built just a stone's throw from my parents' home, on the south coast and near to the beach. The opportunity to live nearer to my parents, have their support with our growing family, and give the children a childhood like my own growing up by the beach was a dream come true. So in June 1998 we moved to West Sussex, and the village and place I had always called home.

Life was hectic, with two school-age children, an endless round of after-school activities like swimming and dance classes, a young baby that hardly ever slept, and now I was pregnant again with my fourth baby. I managed to maintain a much-modified fitness routine throughout this time by attending a gym in the local leisure centre, as well as being active with my children by cycling, swimming and walking together as much as possible.

My fourth baby, and second daughter, Saffron, arrived after a vaginal breech birth on 25 April 1999. I stayed in hospital for a mere six hours after her delivery before being discharged to go home. But during this brief stay we were visited by a constant stream of medics, midwives and student midwives. No one could remember another baby being born via a planned vaginal breech delivery, and everyone wanted to meet us. It gave me a newfound sense of awe for my body. I think a big part of having a fit and active lifestyle is being finely tuned to your body. It gives you confidence in what your body is capable of – like giving birth to a breech baby – but you also recognise when something doesn't feel quite right. On a small scale this can mean recognising the early warning signs of a cold or an infection, but equally it could be something of potential significance, like ongoing abdominal pain, that pushes you to seek early medical advice.

With a newborn, a nine-month-old baby and two young children to ferry to and from school, it was challenging to find time for myself, let alone to exercise. My main form of exercise in the first few weeks was pushing Gabriel and Saffron in a double buggy and taking them for long power walks on the beach. But once the early postnatal weeks had passed, I knew I needed more options to train at home effectively, around nap times and in the evenings. I purchased a treadmill and some light dumbbells and started to exercise at home. Although the treadmill expired a few years ago, 25 years on, these same dumbbells are still used to this day in my personal training studio. Which really illustrates how key pieces of good-quality fitness equipment are a sensible long-term investment.

By the time Saffron was a few months old I had rejoined the gym in the local leisure centre. My training was consistent, but I didn't know anything about exercise science at the time and was simply following a basic routine. The significant turning point in my training came when I joined a new purpose-built gym, Fitness First, in 2001.

Fitness First was by far the biggest, most well-equipped gym I'd ever belonged to. The ground floor was mostly dedicated to an extensive range of cardiovascular equipment, including bikes, treadmills, rowing machines, steppers and elliptical trainers. The first floor had a spinning studio, class studio and full range of resistance machines and free weights with squat racks, benches, Olympic bars and weight plates. A number of self-employed personal trainers worked in the gym, and although I didn't really understand the full benefits of working with a personal trainer (PT), I had a vague idea they might help me understand how to use some of the new equipment I hadn't encountered before. So, I signed up to work with a PT there, Steve, a graduate with a sports science degree who had extensive experience as a strength coach working with the Olympic sailing squad whilst at university. The impact Steve had on my training, my education and understanding about fitness, and determining a new direction for my career, was enormous.

I always remember one of the early conversations I had with Steve. He'd just designed my first training programme, having carried out an initial assessment and gained a better understanding of my main goals. One of my goals, incidentally, was to get muscles like Madonna. So I looked at this training programme and asked him how many days a week I needed to do it for. He said three. Then I asked him how long I'd need to carry on strength training for, to which he replied, 'forever'. This was news to me. Up until this point I hadn't really grasped that fitness is a lifelong journey. I had imagined a training programme was just about getting me from A to B and that would be it; I'd arrive at a destination and I'd stay there.

While working with Steve over the coming months I started to appreciate the benefits of programme design, training cycles, exercise technique and some of the principles of exercise science. In all the years I'd been exercising this was the first time, at the age of 38, that I was making significant progress in my training. I was getting stronger month by month with strength training and achieving a faster running pace.

Steve had taught me so much and ignited my interest in learning more. So I enrolled on a personal training course to further my knowledge, with a vague idea that I might want to teach others at some point.

I started taking my running a little more seriously as well and I entered my first local 10k race in May 2002. I didn't know it at the time, but I was also pregnant with my fifth baby, which I discovered a couple of weeks later. Steve supported my aim to be fit and active and to continue to train throughout my pregnancy. He adapted my programme through each trimester, and during the process I gained valuable first-hand experience of how many exercises can be modified.

The birth of my fifth and final baby, a boy called Jasper, was a little scary. His was another planned home birth, but he was a big baby and became stuck during the delivery. Shoulder dystocia is an obstetric emergency and complication of vaginal delivery in which the baby's shoulder gets caught above the mother's pubic bone. Luckily for both Jasper and me a combination of my change of birth position and the skill of the midwives ensured his safe delivery.

Life became even more complicated with five young children, having school and nurseries to get to and from, as well as after-school activities. In the early weeks, Steve visited me at home a few times, to discuss, design and guide me through a plan for postnatal exercise recovery. Then, when Jasper was a few months old, I found a child-minder for a couple of mornings a week so I could continue my fitness studies and return to the gym.

Having attained a good overall level of fitness before my fifth pregnancy, and been able to maintain it, I was able to return to my previous level of fitness after a few months by following a structured plan. At 40 years old, despite having a young baby, I felt I was the fittest and healthiest I'd ever been.

Juggling lots of demands on my time was challenging, but being physically fit gave me the energy and enthusiasm to manage them. By this time I'd learned to use free weights effectively and was trying to balance my desire to build more muscle along with taking running more seriously. I'd started to enter races, tried a couple of different running clubs, and sometimes paired up with a running partner from the gym or one of the clubs. By the time I'd run a couple of half marathons I knew I wanted to challenge myself with a full marathon distance.

So, in 2007, at the age of 44, I entered my first London Marathon. A friend's young son had been diagnosed with cancer. I applied for a charity place with CLIC Sargent, now known as Young Lives vs Cancer. It seemed like the most practical, and only realistic way that I could help and show my support was by raising money for the charity that was helping my friend and her son. Training for a marathon is very time-consuming, but strength training is also important. During this time my focus was on maintaining leg strength, for endurance and to reduce the risk of injury.

April 22, 2007, was one of the warmest London Marathon days on record, with a temperature that peaked at 22.2 degrees Celsius. It was a beautiful day for running, and unlike some runners I tend to perform better in warmer conditions than colder ones. I felt absolutely elated when I crossed the finish line with my running partner.

I'd run 26.2 miles over 5 hours without stopping, raised an enormous sum of money for CLIC Sargent, and I felt invincible.

I'd proved to myself I was capable; I'd struggled with a couple of niggly injuries, including a knee issue, and I wanted to get back to strength training in earnest. I thought I'd never run another marathon again.

Caught up in the euphoria of running the marathon, I decided to enter the 2008 ballot, not expecting to gain a place. Only I did get offered a place, which, knowing how hard they are to come by, meant I had to run the London Marathon for two years in a row!

Although I wasn't expected to raise money for charity this time around, I thought, if I'm running 26 miles again, I need a strong incentive and reason to keep going. I decided to support a local charity, The Sussex Snowdrop Trust, who provide 'Nursing Care at Home' for local children who have a life-threatening or terminal illness. So, in 2008 I ran my second London Marathon. The weather was in complete contrast to the previous year. This time it didn't stop raining! It was a relief when I finally made it over the finish line – 10 minutes faster than the previous year – especially as I'd developed plantar fasciopathy earlier in my training cycle and was only able to continue running with the aid of a steroid injection in my heel.

When Jasper started school I was able to start taking my work as a fitness coach more seriously. I worked with Steve as a PT in Fitness First. Although this was great experience, I knew it wasn't a good fit for me in the longer term. I was aware from the other mums I'd meet on the school run, and friends and family, that lots of people have a desire to improve their health and fitness, but not everyone feels comfortable in a gym. Plus, some women really prefer a greater level of privacy and feel self-conscious in a gym environment. So, I bought some more pieces of fitness equipment, to add to the treadmill and weights I already had, and started to see clients in my own house. Alongside this I started up an outdoor postnatal fitness class for mums with babies in buggies.

The space I was using at home for training clients was expanding, and my knowledge and experience as a coach was growing. So when a tutor and assessor position arose with one of the UK's leading fitness training providers in 2010, I knew this was an opportunity I wanted to explore. I had previous experience in teaching and delivering courses to adult learners both as a training manager for a large retailer before Tobias was born, and as an antenatal teacher with the NCT. The courses I delivered were taught at the weekend, and I balanced my work with clients and childcare duties during the week alongside this.

As well as teaching students embarking on a career in fitness, taking PT sessions with clients and running my postnatal fitness classes, I was still firmly focused on my own fitness training goals. Running was still a passion, but I wanted a new challenge, so in 2011, at the age of 48, I set my sights on competitive bodybuilding. One of the reasons I wanted to test myself in this way was to understand the discipline required but also the difficulty of stripping body fat whilst retaining lean muscle. I've maintained a steady body weight throughout my life, I didn't have first-hand experience of what it's like to try to reduce body fat before I competed. Weight loss, which is more accurately described as reducing levels of body fat, is a common goal for many clients. Putting myself through this process was a real eye-opener into how hard it is to drop even a small amount of body fat, let alone the several kilograms that many people often want to lose.

Bodybuilding also satisfied my desire to focus on strength training. But I was already lean, and with the benefit of hindsight I would have benefited from spending a couple of years building more muscle, and adding size, before trying to strip body fat. By the time I stepped on stage for my first competition a year later, in June 2012, a regional qualifier for a national bodybuilding competition, I was the leanest I'd ever been. My face looked gaunt as a result, but I placed and was invited to compete in the finals. I competed in a drug-free tested federation, which means the competitors are tested to ensure they aren't taking performance-enhancing drugs (PEDs). As a natural athlete, and someone who does not take PEDs, I wanted a level playing field when I stood on stage, and for my physique to be judged alongside other natural athletes. I didn't place in the finals of this national natural bodybuilding competition, which took place in the September, but I'd been bitten by the bug and decided to compete again in several other competitions.

I won the next competition I took part in. Stage performance was of greater importance in this competition, alongside physique. Although I don't think I was the most muscular, I knew something about stage presence, dance and performance. I performed my routine to 'All That Jazz', and I think this is what swung it for me. I continued to compete in several bodybuilding and physique-type contests for two years.

However, there was a side to competing that increasingly concerned me as someone who has always focused on a 'health first' approach to fitness and exercise. Bodybuilding competitions primarily focus on aesthetics, muscle size, symmetry and definition. Health, athleticism, performance and function aren't the focus, and unfortunately competing can act as a catalyst for issues like body dysmorphia, disordered eating and spending hours in the gym forgoing all other life-enhancing activities. The emphasis on leanness for competition and stripping body fat, then bulking in the off season, 'cheat day' meals and the knock-on disruption to a woman's menstrual cycle, is hardly a recipe for good health. Although I have never had an eating disorder and have always enjoyed a reasonably healthy relationship with food and my body, I realised competing comes at a price for many competitors. It was time for me to step away from the stage.

It seems completely insane to me now that I was competing while I was going through menopause. I experienced some disruption to my monthly cycle during this time, but I still don't know to this day how much of this was related to my low body fat levels (required for competing) and how much was down to perimenopause symptoms.

There was scant education for women on the topic of menopause in 2012. It's only been through extending my own knowledge as a fitness professional in this field in the intervening years that I'm able to look back at my own menopause journey and make sense of some of my experiences and symptoms.

The minute I stopped competing, at the age of 52, and from what I understood about menopause, I knew I needed to maintain a focus on exercise and activities to support my long-term health. The change in hormones at menopause puts women at increased risk of cardiovascular disease and loss of bone density leading to osteoporosis. So,

I carried on with a bodybuilding-type approach to my strength training and a mixture of cardiovascular activities, including running and cycling, for my heart health.

Out of nowhere I started to experience an issue with my left shoulder. I finally realised this was more than a passing problem when I was unable to reach behind my back to do up my bra and couldn't put my arm into a sleeve. Adhesive capsulitis, or frozen shoulder as it's commonly referred to, is a painful restrictive condition especially prevalent in women of menopause age. I tried rest, stretching, physio, strengthening exercises, but nothing made a difference and the pain at night was hideous. As training my upper body was so problematic during this time, I ended up doing a lot of 'leg day' workouts. Eventually I saw an orthopaedic surgeon for further tests, scans, X-rays and a steroid injection into the shoulder (which didn't make a difference), but after two years of struggling and pain the only real option I had was surgery – known as capsular release with subacromial decompression. Thankfully, this was successful, although unfortunately the surgery had to be repeated two years later when my shoulder seized up for a second time.

I continued to train clients from my home studio throughout these years, but when my eldest son left home for good and my daughter started university, it provided an opportunity to expand the studio training space and add to the equipment I had available.

Although I was happy working with a variety of clients, in my home studio I'd primarily focused on training female clients. Training and education as a personal trainer are never complete, we must constantly update our skills and knowledge and take specialist courses on subjects that are particularly relevant to the type of clients we work with. During this time, I was updating my own knowledge by attending menopause conferences and taking courses in female health topics.

The expansion of my studio space was coupled with a small rebrand and the studio became known as Her Garden Gym. Then in December 2016 I started my Instagram account @hergardengym. Initially, this was to promote my personal training services to local clients, and I had no idea how my account and my fitness career would evolve in the years to follow.

Then the global pandemic hit, and everything changed.

On 23 March 2020, Prime Minister Boris Johnson announced a nationwide lockdown to curb a widening outbreak of COVID-19 in the United Kingdom. Many businesses and other sectors were closed, and people were instructed to work from home. Gyms had to shut, and personal trainers like me were no longer able to work with clients face-to-face. Small gym equipment like handheld weights, kettlebells and medicine balls sold out overnight, as people rushed to buying anything they could to exercise at home.

Across the world there was much uncertainty, humanity was being challenged in numerous ways. Staying at home was restrictive and very difficult for many people, but for others it felt comforting and safe. Avid gym goers and those who enjoyed activities like park runs or various sports that involved other people, missed their regular training routine. Even those who'd never exercised before, or had little fitness experience, suddenly became interested in movement and activity to break up the boredom of life in lockdown and working from home.

Many trainers, like me, pivoted to training clients online. It was a time of great ingenuity, utilising technology to coach our clients remotely, and overcoming barriers to training at home like lack of equipment and small spaces to work out in. I started to share more information, education and short home workouts via my Instagram account, and via my Facebook group I shared daily free workouts.

I was truly thankful to have access to a wide range of equipment in my own studio for my personal use, and the beach to run on during this time. But, like many other gym goers, I missed the extensive range of strength-training equipment available in the gym. Extending the range of strength-training equipment I had at home was something I would revisit when the UK finally came out of lockdown in July 2021.

During the UK lockdowns, and as part of my Facebook group, I ran a challenge aimed at supporting the group members to be active. Part of the challenge included tallying up how many miles we walked, cycled or ran each week. I did the challenge as well, and my regular weekly mileage was over 100 miles. I started to experience a knee niggle again, which felt like the same issue I'd been aware of when I'd run the marathon 14 years earlier. I backed off the mileage, thinking this was probably the root of the problem, but my knee grumbled on.

This wasn't the only joint issue I was experiencing, though.

As non-emergency, or non-Covid-related medical treatment was nearly impossible to obtain during the various lockdowns we had in 2020 and 2021, I couldn't see anyone about a developing problem I had in my right shoulder. I recognised the signs immediately and knew I was experiencing another frozen shoulder. I had been warned about this, as women who experience a frozen shoulder are at an increased risk of developing the condition again in their other shoulder. This occurs in about 10 per cent of people within five to seven years of the first frozen shoulder. Just my luck to be part of the 10 per cent.

By the end of 2021, and after failing to resolve my frozen shoulder with conservative treatment, I underwent shoulder surgery for a third time, albeit the first time on my right shoulder. The inflammation, capsular constriction and shoulder impingement in my right shoulder was worse than it had been in my left shoulder. The surgery wasn't exactly an overnight success, and I was in worse pain for the first twelve weeks post-surgery than I had experienced prior to surgery. Eventually, my consultant decided a steroid injection would assist my post-op recovery. Thankfully, this did make a significant difference in reducing the pain and helped me to continue to work on my physio and post-op rehabilitation exercises.

No one undergoes surgery lightly, and there are always pros and cons to weigh up. I'm still not sure, three years later, if this was the right option. It seemed like the only option at the time, though, and at any point in life we can only hope to make the best decision we can in the moment and with all the information then available to us. To this day my right shoulder remains something of an issue. I don't have full range of movement – although that's not completely unusual following surgery – and I am not pain-free. I think this is important for you to know. Whilst the whole premise of this book is about how active ageing can have a positive influence on health span, many of us will face challenges to our health as we grow older. Being active doesn't necessarily mean having no issues to work around. Active ageing is about supporting the healthiest version of you.

During one of my physiotherapy sessions following my shoulder surgery, I asked my physio to carry out an assessment on my knees as well, as I'd been experiencing some discomfort from them. She carried out a rudimentary assessment and based on her findings she recommended a referral to an orthopaedic surgeon who specialised in sports-related injuries to the knee. There's a popular phrase that we use in personal training: 'Assess don't guess', which underlines the importance of fitness tests and assessments to aid safe and appropriate exercise prescription. I apply the same principle to injuries or physical issues. If it's a problem that lingers and starts to impact our lives, it's time to seek an assessment. I already had my suspicions as to what the issue in my knees could be, especially my right knee. To make some informed decisions about my training, though, I needed a definitive diagnosis. After meeting with an orthopaedic surgeon and describing my symptoms, I had an MRI scan. The scan confirmed my worst suspicions – I had osteoarthritis.

Cartilage acts as a cushion and shock absorber at the end of bones, and osteoarthritis (OA) is a degenerative joint condition that occurs when this cartilage wears away and deteriorates, causing pain, stiffness and swelling. Osteoarthritis is most common in the knee joint and affects women more than men. In my case the cartilage had deteriorated to nothing, and I have what's referred to as 'bone-on-bone' knee osteoarthritis. Whilst there is no cure for osteoarthritis, the condition can be managed with exercise and medicinal pain relief.

The orthopaedic surgeon discussed my lifestyle with me, my activity level and the sort of exercise I enjoy. As someone who specialises in working with athletes, he was extremely sympathetic but also reassuring about the important role that exercise plays in the management of knee OA. He identified a few exercises that were best avoided and would likely exacerbate knee pain and swelling. He had no concerns about running on flat surfaces but advised me it would be best to avoid running on hills or uneven surfaces. Lunges and open-chain exercises (where the foot is free and not fixed or in contact with the ground or an object) were out, but split squats and closed-chain exercises would be okay.

We also discussed injection therapy to reduce knee pain, maintain function and postpone, if not eliminate, the need for surgery. After three shoulder surgeries, with the third feeling less than 100 per cent successful, I was of the opinion that surgery was not something I'd want to consider – at least not until, or if, my knee became unbearably painful.

So, I opted for a hyaluronic acid (HA) injection in my knee. HA acts as a lubricant, offloading the articular lining damaged by knee osteoarthritis. It can preserve knee function and reduce pain in some people. My experience of this is that you don't feel an immediate benefit and dramatic difference; it works slowly and reduces rather than eliminates discomfort. The effects of HA wear off within a year, and by around nine months post injection I noticed a grinding, gritty feeling in my knee again. A further injection one year later helped reduce this. At the time of writing, I am hopeful I can continue with these annual injections and avoid surgery.

At the start of my sixties, despite living with osteoarthritis and a history of shoulder surgeries, I was still able to make strength gains in the gym and was ecstatic to set a new deadlift record of 112.5kg with the trap bar. As I was making gains in my strength and physical achievements in my fifties and sixties, interest was growing in the content I was sharing on social media. This response reinforces how important it is to have active-ageing role models who challenge the poor expectations we may have about our physical capabilities as we grow older. I, too, benefit from this, as I seek out social media accounts of women who are physically active, taking part in sports or regular gym goers who are 10–20 years older than me. The old adage *when we see it we can be it* rings true when it comes to exercise and ageing.

However, I was about to face my biggest challenge to date, in the summer of 2024, when disaster struck.

Whilst on holiday I suffered a serious injury, fracturing my left wrist in a freak accident falling backwards from a raised patio area. Apart from being an incredibly painful injury, I was devastated and immediately recognised the impact this would have on my everyday life and my training. It would take me months of hand therapy and, I believe, discovering the benefits of cross-education to work my way back to my previous level of strength pre-injury. (The cross-education phenomena is the strength that can be gained in an opposite limb through unilateral strength training.[1] During the weeks and months when I could not lift weights with my injured left hand, I continued to strength train using my right hand. In this way I believe that I attenuated the loss of muscular strength in my left arm. Some research suggests that had I stopped all upper body strength training, a 28 per cent muscle loss would have occurred in my injured arm in the first four weeks alone.)

My personal fitness journey continues to evolve. You could be forgiven for thinking that with three shoulder surgeries, a diagnosis of osteoarthritis and a wrist fracture that I need to take it easy. But this idea that we will experience slow physical decline as we age, and that's our destiny, needs to be challenged. Poor functional ability for day-to-day life is not an inevitability of older age, but it is an inevitable outcome when we don't engage in physical activity. It's one of the reasons I've written this book. I want more women to enjoy a better quality of life as they grow older. Having an active-ageing approach will enable you to have a huge influence on your future health trajectory and reject the low expectations that your grandparents and great-grandparents had for their older age. I've combined my years of experience as a personal trainer with my lifelong journey in fitness, and the physical challenges I have faced along the way, to bring you this definitive guide to active ageing. In my sixties I am walking the talk, I'm not merely theorising on the benefits of active ageing, I am living it day by day and I want you to enjoy the same benefits and live it with me too.

This book is about showing you how we can enjoy physical activity, deal with challenges along the way, and age better as a result.

HOW TO USE THIS BOOK

I invite you to come on a journey with me as we explore ageism and attitudes to growing older, some of the factors that influence how we age and what we can do about them, the challenging changes that many of us will encounter in midlife, and the impact of menopause on long-term health and ageing.

All these topics will help you understand the things you can't control – like the fact of growing older – but more importantly the things you do have some influence over – like *how* you grow older.

We will look at what fitness means and define it so that you can consider what aspects of fitness are important to you. I recommend you start to think about this in terms of short- and longer-term goals. My clients' short-term goals have included taking part in a park run, going on a five-day hiking trip with fitter friends, and being able to enjoy gardening without experiencing back pain. Consider your longer-term goals, too. What would you like your life to look like 10, 15, 20 years from now? What do you do today that will still be important to you in years to come? If you currently enjoy long country walks with your partner (or a dog!), do you want to be able to continue doing so in your eighties or nineties? What are your living arrangements now, do you see this changing or remaining the same when you are older? Is overseas travel important to you?

Your goals are likely to change over time as well, so come back to them regularly and review them. Focusing on consistency and establishing a regular exercise habit is a realistic goal for many people at the start of their fitness journey. Your initial goal could be as simple as committing to and completing the recommended weekly plans in this book. It doesn't matter if you are new to exercise, haven't exercised for a while or are a seasoned pro, there is something in this book for everyone.

The fitness section covers everything you need to know about addressing the eleven components of fitness, which includes five health-related and six skill-related components, that we will explore in the next chapter. Breaking down fitness into these components helps bring clarity to what it means to be 'fit'. We will look at pelvic health and its relevance to exercise, as well as ageing and overall well-being. If you plan to exercise at home, we will be covering what equipment I recommend for the workouts contained in this book, any relevant health and safety considerations and the importance of reviewing your current health status before you embark on a new fitness regime.

There are fun fitness challenges throughout, as well as reference tables for common fitness tests, which you may want to try to establish as a baseline and repeat at regular intervals to monitor your progress.

Included in this book is a comprehensive exercise library with step-by-step instructions and illustrations throughout, so that if an exercise is unfamiliar you will understand what it is, the benefits of it, and how to do it.

I have provided a range of different workouts to support your cardiovascular health, strength and conditioning, flexibility and mobility, agility and balance. You'll also find some short-exercise 'snack' sessions, each of which take no longer than 10 minutes and will help inject some movement into your busiest days. There are weekly plans from beginner through to intermediate – both are twelve weeks long and divided into two phases.

You'll find modifications and adaptations of the exercises throughout so that you can work around any temporary or longer-term physical restrictions you might have, and we will look at some specific prehabilitation and rehabilitation exercises for common musculoskeletal problems that women experience in midlife.

The nutrition chapters in this book cover some basic facts about food, including macronutrients and micronutrients and how dietary intake influences health, function and your wellbeing. We will look at what constitutes a healthy diet, as well as factors that influence body weight and weight management as we grow older. Together we will explore dietary patterns of eating and the scientific evidence behind them, to support healthier ageing. We will also look at how some dietary strategies are helping in the management of common health issues associated with increasing age.

Throughout my book you will find references to the latest research on many of the topics covered. If you want to dive deeper, you'll be able to look up these references and read more on the areas that interest you the most. I've included a separate glossary as well, to demystify common fitness terms and words that you may come across.

You can dip in and out of this book, reading whichever sections interest you the most, skip straight to the workouts, or read it cover to cover. It's up to you. I personally would recommend you read the whole book to fully appreciate what happens to our bodies during the ageing process, the challenges we may face, and why resilience, persistence and consistency are your greatest allies on your active-ageing journey.

Influencing the future of your health trajectory is at the heart of my book. I hope you read it, enjoy it, then take action to lengthen your health span.

CHAPTER 1

WHAT IS PHYSICAL FITNESS?

When we think about what fitness means to us, we probably all imagine something slightly different. Fitness is defined in the dictionary as 'the condition of being physically strong and healthy'. Olympic athletes, elite marathon runners and professional footballers are examples of peak physical fitness in different sports. We may not aspire to or believe this level of 'fitness' is achievable for us, though – park runners, gym goers and attendees of group fitness classes are more relatable examples of fitness for most of us.

But clearly there's a big difference between someone who competes in the 10,000-metre track run at the Olympic Games and someone who takes part in an organised 10k running race. If speed was the only measure of fitness, it would be easy to understand who is the 'fittest'.

In bodybuilding, competitors are judged based on their physiques, including muscle mass, definition, symmetry and balance. Female bodybuilding competition categories include bikini, fitness, figure, physique and wellness, in recognition of the different training goals, genetics and type of competitor. Bodybuilders spend many hours in the gym, lifting weights and sculpting their physiques. They pay careful attention to their diet and nutrition to support muscle retention and growth, and to reduce body fat. Does lifting weights in the gym, following a careful diet and achieving a particular aesthetic indicate a level of fitness, though?

And if bodybuilding isn't your cup of tea, what about yogis? You need flexibility, balance and strength for challenging yoga exercises such as King Pigeon, headstands and Crow Pose. Are the people who can perform the hardest and most advanced yoga poses 'fitter' than those who enjoy chair yoga?

These examples – speed, muscularity, flexibility – demonstrate how 'fitness' can mean something different to all of us, which is potentially very confusing! But these examples are merely components of fitness, and not the whole picture.

Physical fitness can be better understood by recognising different components. It is widely accepted that there are 11 components of fitness that can be broken down into five health-related components and six skill-related components.

Health-related components

1. Body composition: The proportion of bone, muscle and fat in the body.
2. Cardiovascular fitness: The ability of the heart and blood vessels to supply nutrients and oxygen to tissues and muscles throughout the body.
3. Flexibility: The ability of muscles, joints and soft tissues to move through an unrestricted, pain-free range of motion.
4. Muscular endurance: The ability of a muscle or group of muscles to exert force against a load, consistently and repetitively.
5. Strength: The amount of force a muscle or group of muscles can exert against a resistance.

Skill-related components

1. Agility: The ability to move rapidly and change direction.
2. Balance: The ability to maintain control and stability of the body, over a base of support, when stationary and during movement.
3. Coordination: The ability to control and use two or more body parts together.
4. Power: The ability to generate maximal force quickly, combining speed and strength.
5. Reaction time: The ability to respond quickly to a stimulus.
6. Speed: The ability to move the whole body, or a limb, quickly.

If we assessed the 10k runners, bodybuilders and yogis on the health- and skill-related components of fitness, each would differ. We'd expect the runners to have a good level of cardiovascular fitness, the bodybuilders to have the highest proportion of muscle, and the yogis to be the most flexible. But none of them might be assessed as 'good' in all 11 components of fitness.

Based on these described components of fitness, it becomes clear that being good at one or two components does not indicate overall level of fitness. Maintaining an awareness of these 11 components of fitness, and including them in daily life as well as structured physical activity, might seem like the obvious way to get 'fit', but is it realistic to be competent or 'good' at all 11 components of fitness, and is it possible to work on improving all of them at the same time?

Triathlons, pentathlons, heptathlons and decathlons are demanding events for athletes. They are great examples of sports where multiple components of fitness are tested. But even at Olympic level it's not unusual for athletes to be stronger in one discipline than another. In a triathlon some triathletes may excel at swimming but can lack endurance on the bike. Other triathletes are excellent runners but are not as proficient at swimming.

If highly trained athletes have weaknesses and strengths when tested across several disciplines, it's reasonable to conclude that most of us will struggle to excel in every component of fitness – but we can certainly aim for a more rounded approach to our fitness, like these athletes.

So let's look at these components of fitness in greater detail, and how they may alter or be impacted by age.

Body composition

The proportions of fat, bone and muscle in the body change throughout an individual's lifespan, and ageing is typically associated with changes to body composition such as a decrease in muscle mass and an increase in body fat levels. Muscle and fat distribution can also change according to age and gender. Alongside this, bone density typically peaks by the time we reach our late twenties then it starts to decrease. The proportion of fat, bone and muscle in the body has a direct effect on health, so as an active ager we will be focusing on optimising body composition to support healthier ageing.

Fat

Fat in a human body can be broken down into essential fat and body fat. Essential fat is present in numerous organs throughout the body and assists with normal bodily functions. Body fat acts as fat storage and is found around the organs (visceral) and under the skin (subcutaneous).

Non-essential body fat often increases with age, with decreasing levels of physical activity, combined with surplus energy intake (from food and drinks). Hormonal changes at menopause also alter fat distribution, increasing the likelihood that excess fat will be stored around the abdomen, rather than on the hips and thighs.

Visceral fat is non-essential fat, and an excess of this increases the risk of health issues and chronic diseases. Maintaining a physically active lifestyle as we age can contribute to keeping body fat levels in an optimal range, reducing risks to health.

Bone

Bone mass is the total mass of skeletal bone in the body. The terms bone mass and bone density are often used interchangeably, but they mean different things. Bone mass is the weight of all the skeletal bone in your body, which typically increases during childhood and peaks when you reach full height. Bone density refers to the amount of bone mineral contained within bone; a higher bone density indicates better bone strength, a lower bone density indicates holes within the bones, making them more fragile and at risk of breakage.

Although there's no absolute consensus as to at what age peak mineral bone density is reached, it is widely believed that it is attained somewhere between the early to late twenties. In one study of 18,713 youths, bone mineral density was measured across three skeletal sites (femoral neck, hip and lumbar spine). The study revealed peak femoral neck, total hip and lumbar spine bone mineral density were respectively 20.5 years, 21.2 years and 23.6 years in males, and 18.7 years, 19.0 years and 20.1 years in females.[1]

Childhood, adolescence and early adulthood is the time when we can have the greatest impact on attaining peak bone density, mostly through diet and exercise. Bone density can also be negatively impacted through lifestyle choices such as smoking, excess alcohol consumption, poor nutrition and inactivity. Once peak bone density has been reached, and by the time we reach our forties, bone density starts to decrease.

Bone continues a process of self-regeneration, known as remodelling, throughout our lifespan. Remodelling is where old bone is replaced with new bone, through which a bone fracture repairs and heals. But as we grow older greater bone resorption takes place, and less bone formation occurs, leading to a decrease in bone density. So by the time you reach your seventieth birthday your bone mass may have decreased by as much as 30–40 per cent.

A decrease in bone density leads to weak and fragile bones, with an increased risk of fracture. This is a potential problem for all older adults but especially for women, who have smaller bones than men. In addition, the hormonal changes associated with menopause lead to a rapid decrease in bone density in the first five years following menopause. The average decrease in bone density is thought to be in the region of 10 per cent at this time, but some women may experience as much as 10–20 per cent decrease in the five years after menopause.[2] As a result, osteopenia, where bone mineral density is lower than the normal range for age, can develop.

The rate of bone loss in adults over the age of 40 can be slowed through diet and exercise. This is especially important for women in the peri- to post-menopause years, to mitigate against the hormonal changes that increase bone loss. Osteopenia can develop into osteoporosis without taking the appropriate steps, including diet, exercise and treatment. Osteoporosis is more serious than osteopenia, as it's characterised by low bone density with a heightened risk of a bone fracture occurring. Osteoporosis is often only suspected, and diagnosed, when a fracture has occurred. My doctor referred me for a bone density scan, also known as a DEXA scan, following my wrist fracture. The results of my scan showed that I do not have osteoporosis but worldwide, one in three women and one in five men over the age of 50 will experience a bone fracture due to osteoporosis. These statistics for women worsen with each decade so that osteoporosis affects a tenth of women aged 60, a fifth of women aged 70, two-fifths of women aged 80 and two-thirds of women aged 90.[3]

Two forms of exercise are associated with stimulating bone formation: weight-bearing exercise and strength and resistance-type exercises. Exercises to support bone health form an important part of our active-ageing strategy, and we'll be exploring these in the workout section. Nutrition is also critical to bone health, and we'll be looking at nutritional recommendations for healthier bones within the nutrition section.

Muscle

The body has three different types of muscle: skeletal muscle, smooth muscle and cardiac muscle.

Skeletal muscle

Skeletal muscles are part of the musculoskeletal system and work with bones, tendons and ligaments, supporting the body and being responsible for voluntary movement. Skeletal muscles are comprised of individual muscle fibres known as slow-twitch type I and fast-twitch type II. Fast-twitch type II muscle fibres are further divided into Type IIx and Type IIa. Slow-twitch muscle fibres are smaller, slow to fatigue and are necessary for activities like walking and endurance events, as well as maintaining posture. Fast-twitch muscle fibres are bigger, quicker to fatigue and needed for explosive movement and activities like sprinting or jumping.

All skeletal muscles are a mixture of fast- and slow-twitch, although the proportion of each can vary between individuals. Less-athletic people may have an even balance between fast- and slow-twitch, whereas the differences between the proportion of slow- to fast-twitch muscles are more likely in elite-level athletes. For example, endurance sports athletes – like marathon runners – can have a higher proportion of slow-twitch muscles, whereas athletes with explosive power – like sprinters – may have a higher proportion of fast-twitch muscles.

Muscle mass decreases with age, and the proportion of fast- to slow-twitch muscle fibres changes as fast-twitch convert to slow-twitch. As fast-twitch muscle fibres are bigger than slow-twitch muscle fibres this can still result in the loss of lean muscle and changes to body composition. Loss of lean muscle can also affect daily function and independence in older age.

Strength training can help combat this age-related decrease in muscle mass, and explosive exercises can aid the retention of fast-twitch muscles. This is why our active-ageing strategy incorporates a range of strength exercises as well as explosive strength exercises.

Smooth muscle

Smooth muscle is a type of muscle that contracts without voluntary control. It's referred to as smooth because it lacks the striations found in skeletal and cardiac muscle. Smooth muscle forms the walls in internal organs such as the digestive tract, liver, pancreas and bladder, and the blood vessels of arteries and veins, as well as glands. The expansion and contraction of smooth muscle propels the food you eat, your blood and fluids throughout the body. As an involuntary muscle you have no control over how it works – you don't have to think about how your food is propelled to your stomach and intestines for digestion, or how your blood flows around your body, it just happens.

Cardiac muscle

Cardiac muscle lines the walls of the heart. It is only found in the heart and, like skeletal muscle, it is striated. Cardiac muscle performs involuntary contractions, rhythmically, which keep the heart pumping and create your heartbeat. The contract and release of this cardiac muscle pumps blood, which then travels around the cardiovascular system.

The speed of cardiac muscle contractions, and how fast your heart beats, can be influenced by various factors. At rest, and when physical demands on the body are low, the heart rate slows, but during activity the heart rate increases. Healthier individuals usually have a lower resting heart rate, of between 60 and 100 BPM, with the lower end being preferable. A high resting heart rate can indicate that the cardiac muscle isn't working efficiently.

During physical exertion the heart rate rises in response to the need to deliver oxygenated blood to working muscles. The more intense an activity, the higher the heart rate will rise. This is a normal response to movement and exercise. You may not even be aware of a small rise in heart rate for lower-intensity movement, such as a gentle walk, whereas if you suddenly need to run for a bus, you will probably notice an increase in breathing and heart rate.

Age can affect how efficiently the heart and the cardiac muscle works. As you get older your heart doesn't have the capacity to beat as fast during physical activity as it did when you were younger.

Heart rate is also influenced by stress, blood pressure, illness, hot and cold weather, caffeine, medications, alcohol and smoking. Temporary elevations in heart rate caused by illness, an emotional response, or hot or cold weather are less problematic to cardiac muscle than a sustained elevation from some of these other factors. Long periods of stress, high blood pressure, excess alcohol intake and smoking can all result in damage to cardiac muscle and heart disease. Family history may also increase your risk of heart disease.

Heart disease is a result of the build-up of fatty deposits, known as plaque, in the coronary arteries. The arteries become stiff and harden, which reduces blood flow to the heart muscle and can weaken and damage it.

The factors that influence cardiac muscle and heart health can be grouped by those that you can influence, known as modifiable risk factors, and those you can't, known as non-modifiable risk factors.

Modifiable risk factors include:
- High blood pressure
- High cholesterol
- Type 2 diabetes
- Smoking
- Body weight
- Sedentary lifestyle
- Physical inactivity

Non-modifiable risk factors include:
- Family history
- Age
- Ethnic background

Our active-ageing strategy can play a significant role in the retention of skeletal muscle and the health of cardiac muscle.

Cardiovascular fitness

Cardiovascular (CV) fitness refers to the ability of the heart and blood vessels to supply nutrients and oxygen to tissues and muscles throughout the body.

Cardiovascular fitness is also referred to as aerobic fitness, or aerobic capacity, and CV. Regular cardiovascular activity helps maintain and improve cardiovascular fitness. This includes any activity that elevates the heart rate. Examples of lower-intensity cardiovascular activities include walking, seated exercise classes, slow dancing, gardening and swimming. Higher-intensity cardiovascular activities include running, circuit training, rowing, burpees and skipping.

Heart rate training zones are used to assess exercise intensity. These zones are calculated based on maximum heart rate and expressed as a percentage. Monitoring heart rate during cardiovascular activity is required for this. A fitness tracker watch is an easy way to monitor heart rate at home for this purpose, although it isn't 100 per cent accurate.

A simple way to calculate your maximum heart rate (MHR) is using the Fox Formula of MHR = 220 − Age. Using this calculation, a woman who is 50 will have a theoretical maximum heart rate of 170 (220 − 50 = 170).

Although this method is simple, it's not very accurate and research has shown a standard deviation of the maximum heart rate equation of 220 − Age in years is +/− 12 beats per minute.[4]

There are many other formulas that can be used to calculate maximum heart rate, including the following two alternatives.

Tanaka formula

The Tanaka formula may be more accurate for women over 40 because the 220 – Age formula is associated with higher errors for older adults.

This formula is 208 – (0.7 × Age), so the maximum heart rate for a 50-year-old woman using this formula is 173.

Gulati formula

The Gulati formula was developed specifically for women after other formulas were shown to consistently overestimate maximum heart rate for women.[5]

This formula is 206 – (0.88 × Age). The maximum heart rate for a 50-year-old woman using this formula is 162.

These three formulas demonstrate a range of theoretical maximum heart rates for a 50-year-old woman as 170, 173 and 162.

You may wish to use the formulas to calculate your own theoretical maximum heart rate ranges. Using one of these will be sufficient to estimate appropriate heart rate training zones, but the only definitive way to establish your actual maximum heart rate is with a field or laboratory test, which can be important for athletes and to maximise performance.

There are five main training zones:

Zone	Intensity	Percentage of HR max
Zone 1	Very light	50–60%
Zone 2	Light	60–70%
Zone 3	Moderate	70–80%
Zone 4	Hard	80–90%
Zone 5	Maximum	90–100%

For example, a 50-year-old woman will have a theoretical maximum heart rate of 170 (220 – 50 = 170), so her training zones would be as follows.

Zone	Intensity	Percentage of HR max
Zone 1	Very light	50–60% of 170 = 85 – 102 bpm
Zone 2	Light	60–70% of 170 = 102 – 119 bpm
Zone 3	Moderate	70–80% of 170 = 119 – 136 bpm
Zone 4	Hard	80–90% of 170 = 136 – 153 bpm
Zone 5	Maximum	90–100% of 170 = 153 – 170 bpm

Our active-ageing strategy incorporates a range of cardiovascular workouts. Heart rate training zones may be something you wish to monitor, but we will also look at other methods so you can pick what's appropriate for you.

Flexibility

The ability of your muscles, joints and soft tissues to move through an unrestricted, pain-free range of motion can be summed up as flexibility.

Having adequate flexibility can improve many activities of daily life, assist in sports performance, reduce the risk of injury and aid posture. Wide differences in levels of flexibility can vary from person to person, but there are optimal ranges that support joint health and ease of movement.

Factors that impact flexibility include injury, damage or disease in the joint and lack of exercise – specifically stretching, age and genetics. The surrounding structures and tissues, muscles, tendons, ligaments and joint capsules can also all affect flexibility.

Restrictions in flexibility can affect cartilage and lead to muscular imbalances as well as stress to surrounding structures. But reduced flexibility, and an inadequate range of movement in a joint, can be improved with regular stretching.

As increasing age can signal a reduction in flexibility, working on maintaining flexibility and mobility is an important aspect of our active-ageing strategy.

Muscular endurance

The ability of a muscle or group of muscles to exert force against a load, consistently and repetitively, is known as muscular endurance.

In activities like running, cycling and swimming a good level of muscular endurance allows for a continuation over an extended period. Triathlons are a good example of this. Muscular endurance is also required when lifting weights for higher numbers of repetitions. In day-to-day life muscular endurance determines how long and how hard you can continue performing a movement, like climbing up several flights of stairs when the lift is out of order.

Muscular endurance, and the ability of your muscles to exert force against a load repeatedly, decreases in age in line with muscle loss. Strength training can combat age-related decline in muscle size and strength, both of which are necessary for muscular endurance. Supporting the retention of muscle size and strength allows specific muscular endurance training to take place.

Muscular endurance is another important component of an active-ageing strategy.

Strength

Strength is the amount of force a muscle or group of muscles can exert against a resistance.

Muscular strength is necessary for day-to-day activities, physical exercise and sports performance. In daily activities muscular strength is needed to walk up a flight of stairs, lift and carry shopping bags, and put a large casserole dish in the oven. Adequate muscular strength allows us to get out of a chair with ease and use the toilet unaided. Body-weight exercises like squats and push-ups require muscular strength, alongside exercises where weights, like dumb-bells and kettlebells, or resistance machines are used.

Muscular strength decreases with age alongside the loss of muscle size, power and changes in muscle fibre. Muscle mass decreases at a rate of between 3 and 8 per cent each decade after the age of 30. This directly impacts the ability of muscle, or a group of muscles, to generate force against a resistance.

In order for a muscle to get stronger it must also increase in size; this is known as hypertrophy. For muscular hypertrophy to occur, muscles must be stimulated via strength training and receive the right nutrients to support growth via diet in the form of adequate protein. Women have less total muscle mass than men and are unable to develop muscles as large as men. This is partly down to lower levels of testosterone in women compared to men, the hormone that helps promote the growth of lean muscle. In one study the biceps of competitive male bodybuilders were found to be twice the size of their female counterparts, even after years of training. So, if getting too muscular is a concern, don't worry, the growth in muscle that women get from strength training is proportionate to their physique.[6]

Strength training is beneficial at any age, but as you grow older it is essential to offset and slow down the rate of loss of muscle size and strength associated with ageing.

This is fundamental to our active-ageing approach, and I will introduce you to some key strength exercises in the workout section (Chapter 8).

There are two conditions that can significantly impact muscle strength, size and endurance, and although they are not a component of fitness, they are relevant to mention here.

Sarcopenia

Sarcopenia is the gradual loss of muscle size and occurs from your thirties onwards.[7] Although you may hear the gradual loss of muscle strength referred to as dynapenia, in studies on ageing and in the literature, sarcopenia is often defined as loss of muscle size and strength, so, for the sake of clarity, I am using this same definition.

Stages of sarcopenia have been classified by the European Working Group on Sarcopenia in Older People as presarcopenia, sarcopenia and severe sarcopenia. Risk factors for sarcopenia include increasing age, gender (higher prevalence in women) and physical inactivity.

Sarcopenia is a major component of frailty, which has a detrimental effect on quality of life and ability to live independently.

Sarcopenic obesity

The prevalence and growth of obesity worldwide, alongside increases in life expectancy, has seen the emergence of a condition known as sarcopenic obesity. This is a relatively new classification in older adults who are characterised by the loss of muscle mass and strength with age, coupled with an increase in body fat. Sarcopenic obesity is associated with an increased risk of cardiovascular disease and mortality.[8]

Agility

A popular definition of agility is the ability to move rapidly and change direction. But an improved definition proposed by Sheppard and Young (2006) states that, '*agility is a rapid whole-body movement with change of velocity or direction in response to a stimulus.*'[9]

Although we often associate agility with sporting activities, it is also relevant for daily life. When a small child suddenly darts across the path of shoppers in a supermarket, the parent may have to react quickly to catch them. Shoppers may also have to react quickly, stepping aside, or changing direction to avoid a collision. When you are walking outside on a rainy day and you suddenly realise you're about to step into a large puddle, you may want to step sideways briskly to avoid getting wet feet. In these examples the stimulus for a change in direction or speed is the child and the puddle. Responding to the stimulus requires cognitive skills including visual processing, perception and anticipation. Responding rapidly to a stimulus also requires fast-twitch muscle fibres, the muscle fibres responsible for fast and explosive movements.

Agility, like other components of fitness, decreases with age as a result of cognitive decline and the reduction in fast-twitch muscle fibres. However, agility can be trained, and incorporating agility exercises into an exercise programme can help offset the natural decline with age.

Balance

Balance can be defined as the ability to maintain control and stability of the body, over a base of support, both when stationary and during movement.

Balance is required in daily life, for actions such as going up and down stairs and getting in and out of a bath, and also for static positions and during dynamic movement. The yoga tree pose is an example of static balance, whereas single leg exercises, like a step up, and activities like walking and running, require dynamic balance. Balance is affected by muscular strength and flexibility, but other issues can have an impact, including visual impairment, hearing loss, some medications, inner ear problems and low blood pressure.

Vision and hearing loss are common in older adults, as well as an increase in prescription medications, so consequently issues with balance as we grow older are not unusual, which is why exercises that assist balance are beneficial.

Coordination

Coordination is the ability to control and use two or more body parts together.

Coordination requires the senses of seeing and hearing and using multiple muscles that result in one coordinated movement. Both fine motor skills and gross motor skills are needed as well. Fine motor skills are required for smaller movements, like holding a small ball, whereas gross motor skills are needed for movements that incorporate bigger muscle groups, such as hopping, skipping and jumping.

Coordination requires movement efficiency; no energy is wasted because the movement is fluid and controlled. It is necessary in sports like badminton and football, as well as activities like writing and getting dressed. In daily life the ability to coordinate body parts is constantly needed for a range of tasks such as walking, picking something up and typing on a laptop or mobile phone.

The ability to coordinate movement and control two or more body parts can diminish with age, alongside changes in muscle strength, the nervous system and the brain. But exercise can help improve coordination and reduce the risk of injury from poor coordination. In one study, exercise programmes that included exercises for coordination reduced rates of falls in older adults by 40 per cent.[10]

Power

Power is defined as the ability to generate maximal force quickly, through combining speed and strength, which are both components of fitness. The ability to generate power is mostly associated with athletic endeavours and sports – Olympic lifts, vertical jumps and kettlebell swings all require power. But power is also something that can be called upon outside of fitness activities, for movements such as getting up off the toilet quickly.

Speed and strength can decrease with age, which has a direct impact on power production, but exercise that incorporates strength and speed, resulting in power, can help offset this decline.

Reaction time

The ability to respond quickly to a stimulus is known as reaction time.

There are many situations when your ability to react quickly is important, whether engaging in a physical activity or day-to-day life. A boxer needs to react quickly to a punch from an opponent, a sprinter needs to react as soon as the start gun is fired, and if you slip on the stairs your speed of reaction can make the difference between grabbing the handrail for support, or injury.

Fast-twitch muscle fibres need to be recruited to quickly react to a stimulus, and experience can influence accuracy in anticipating and reacting accordingly. An older, experienced, racquet sport player can be a fearsome opponent for a younger but inexperienced player.

Reaction times often slow down with age, and this can be impaired by the ability to process and respond to a stimulus, as well as the loss of fast-twitch muscle fibres.[11]

However, the ability to respond quickly to a stimulus can be assisted with training, so that impaired reaction time may be improved.

Speed

Speed is the ability to move the whole body, or a limb, quickly.

It is a common requirement in many sports, including track and field events and team games like hockey and basketball. The ability to move the whole body or just a limb quickly is a skill used in daily life as well, like walking when you're on your lunch break and short on time, or pulling your hand away quickly when you see a door is about to close on it.

The ability to move quickly with speed can diminish with age, so it's another important skill to train in order to offset it.

There is a lot of overlap with these skill-based components of fitness. Many of the exercises I've incorporated in the active-ageing workouts provide a training stimulus for one or more of these skills.

Measuring physical fitness

Various methods are used to measure the health- and skills-related components of physical fitness. Some tests can only be carried out in a clinical setting, monitored by a specialist, or involve invasive or complex methods.

This next section examines a range of fitness tests, some of which you may choose to carry out. Where possible, it can be helpful to undertake some basic tests to establish a baseline, which might also provide valuable information on areas of strengths or weakness, which can aid exercise selection and gauge progress on retesting.

Measuring body composition

There are various methods that can be used to estimate body composition, which include anthropometric, non-invasive measurements of weight, height, abdominal circumference, waist-to-hip ratio and skinfold measurements. Other, more complex, methods include bioelectrical impedance, hydrostatic weighing, dual-energy X-ray absorptiometry, body density and total body water estimates.

Some people find it useful to have an indication of their body composition before they commence a training programme, especially if fat loss is the goal. Others may not feel they want or need this information, and some people with an eating disorder history may find any form of tracking potentially triggering.

The following two methods included here – body mass index and waist-to-hip ratio – are non-invasive and easy to carry out at home, if this is important to you. Although there are flaws and limitations with both, some people find them helpful as a tool to measure progress and observe any changes on retesting.

BMI is particularly controversial, and the UK Parliament Women and Equalities Committee have called on the government to abandon the use of it to determine whether someone's weight is healthy. There are many limitations with BMI, especially when used to make judgements about health. In recognition of this, in 2022 England's National Institute for Health and Care Excellence (NICE) made changes to obesity guidelines, recommending that waist-to-hip ratio be used alongside BMI.[12]

The BMI calculation is included here as reference, and not as an endorsement of this method of assessing body composition.

Body mass index (BMI)

This is calculated by taking body weight in kg and dividing it by height squared. The higher the figure, the more body fat someone may be carrying. However, this is a crude measurement as BMI can't distinguish between weight as body fat or lean muscle. BMI also isn't accurate during pregnancy, with older adults and with very muscular people.

The calculation for BMI = kg/m^2

A BMI of 25.0 or more is classified as 'overweight', while the healthy range is classified as 18.5 to 24.9.

Waist-to-hip ratio (WHR)

A waist-to-hip ratio compares waist measurement to hip measurement. Higher ratios can indicate body fat distribution. When more body fat is stored around the mid-section than the hips it is associated with a higher risk to health.

The calculation for WHR = waist/hips (cm or inches can be used)

According to the World Health Organization (WHO) a WHR higher than 1 can increase the risk of developing some conditions, such as heart disease and type 2 diabetes.[13]

The WHO recommends:

- WHR for women: 0.85 or less
- WHR for men: 0.9 or less

Measuring cardiovascular fitness

Your cardiovascular system supplies blood, which carries oxygen and nutrients throughout your body. When you are engaged in cardiovascular activity, also referred to as aerobic activity, your body has an increased demand for oxygen. The cardiovascular system responds to this by increasing the speed and amount of blood delivered to the body.

The best measurement to assess cardiovascular fitness is a VO_2 max test. VO_2 max is the maximum (max) rate (V) of oxygen (O_2) that your body can use during exercise. Oxygen is a critical part of the respiratory process and breathing. When you breathe in oxygen, your lungs absorb it, then turn it into energy.

A VO_2 max test indicates how much oxygen you are able to utilise during intense exercise. The more oxygen you can use, the more energy you'll be able to generate. A higher VO_2 max means your body can respond well to aerobic activities like running.

Monitoring and improving VO_2 max is important to maximise athletic performance, but you don't have to be an athlete to benefit from improving cardiorespiratory fitness.

A VO_2 max test is normally conducted in a medical facility, or by sports scientists, under strict conditions. A sub-maximal test is more readily available, and a preferred option for most people, as the test is performed below maximum heart rate. This type of test can be conducted in a fitness facility or on a track, overseen by a fitness specialist.

If you wear a fitness tracker watch it may provide you with an estimate of your VO_2 max. This data tends to be more accurate over time, as the tracker builds up a history of your cardiovascular activity and monitors other health markers, such as resting heart rate. Other devices, such as a chest strap that monitors heart rate, can also be utilised for this purpose.

It is also possible carry out your own simple sub-maximal VO_2 max test, known as the Rockport Walk Test

Rockport Walk Test

The Rockport Walk Test requires you to walk as fast as you can (not run) for 1 mile (1.6km) on a level surface, track or treadmill.

You'll need to wear a fitness tracker, or heart rate monitor, and you will require a stopwatch to conduct the test. You'll also need to note your body weight, as this figure is used in the calculation.

Before you begin the test, ensure you conduct a warm-up for 5–10 minutes, focusing on dynamic stretches of the lower body and finishing with some gentle walking to raise the pulse. See the exercise warm-up section on page 146 for suitable examples.

To conduct the Rockport Walk Test
1. When you have completed the warm-up, start your stopwatch and start walking as quickly as you can – do not run.
2. When you have completed the one-mile distance, stop the stopwatch and record the time in decimals.
3. Make a note of your heart rate immediately. You can then use this equation to estimate your VO_2 max or use an online

calculator.[14] Females: VO_2 max (ml/kg/min) = 132.853 − (0.0769 × weight in pounds) − (0.3877 × age) − (3.2649 × mile walk time) − (0.1565 × ending heart rate)[15]

4. Look at your VO_2 max score and grade it against norms for women of your age. I've included the normative data here for males as well.

Normative data (Heywood 2006[16]) for VO_2 max scores for females

Age	20–29	30–39	40–49	50–59	60–69	70–79
Superior	>49	>45	>44	>34	>35	>35
Excellent	44–49	41–45	39–44	31–34	32–35	30–35
Good	40–43	37–40	35–38	29–30	29–31	27–29
Fair	36–39	34–36	32–34	25–28	26–28	24–26

Normative data (Heywood 2006) for VO_2 max scores for males

Age	20–29	30–39	40–49	50–59	60–69	70–79
Superior	>55	<53	>52	>49	>45	>41
Excellent	51–55	48–53	46–52	43–49	39–45	36–41
Good	46–50	44–47	42–45	38–42	35–38	31–35
Fair	42–45	41–43	38–41	35–37	31–34	28–30
Poor	<42	>41	<38	<35	>31	<28

Measuring flexibility

Flexibility, or lack of it, is something we are often more aware of than other components of fitness. We may appreciate that the ability to do the splits requires flexibility, whereas if we can't touch our own toes this indicates a lack of flexibility.

There are numerous tests for flexibility, most will require an assessment with a fitness specialist or a physiotherapist who may use a goniometer (a tool to measure range of motion in a joint).

These are two simple tests you can try at home, though. It's important to warm up thoroughly before conducting these tests, by following the warm-up exercises in the workout section (Chapter 8).

Hamstring flexibility

This test can help assess hamstring flexibility.

1. Lie down on your back, face up.
2. Rest your arms on the floor, at your sides.
3. Extend both legs and straighten them.
4. Gently lift and raise one leg as far as you can, without assistance from your hands, keeping your other leg straight and on the floor. Make a note of the angle (an assistant can be useful for this).
5. Repeat on the other side.

A 90° angle indicates a good level of flexibility. Less than this suggests a restriction in hamstring flexibility.

Shoulder flexibility

This test can assess range of movement and flexibility in the shoulder joint.

1. From a standing position, reach one hand upwards, then over and behind the shoulder.
2. With the other hand, reach backwards. Flexibility is assessed by whether the hands cross over, the fingertips touch, or how far away the fingertips are from each other.
3. Repeat on the other side.

If the fingertips touch, this can indicate a good level of flexibility in the shoulder joint. If they are unable to touch, this suggests a restriction in the shoulder joint.

Measuring strength and endurance

Assessing your current level of muscular strength can provide a useful benchmark. This can be revisited and subsequently retested after a set period to determine the success of a strength-training programme. In the absence of carrying out specific tests, an indication of current muscular strength can be gained based on what weights you are able to work with. For example, in a biceps curl exercise, if you can perform eight repetitions with 4kg dumbbells but no repetitions with a 5kg set then you can simply make a note of this as your starting point.

The following two muscular strength and endurance tests can give you an indication of upper body and lower body strength. Just like the flexibility assessments, it's important to warm up thoroughly before conducting these tests, by following the warm-up exercises in the workout section.

Squat test

This test can evaluate muscular strength and endurance of the legs and lower body. It involves squatting to a chair for as many repetitions as possible.

1. To conduct this test, you will need a solid chair or box that allows your knees to be at right angles when you are seated.
2. Stand in front of the box or chair, feet hip distance apart. Arms can be extended in front of you or remain at your sides.
3. Squat down to the chair, lightly touching your bottom to the chair, and immediately stand up again. Do not rest or sit on the chair during each repetition.
4. If you fail to fully lower yourself, pause to rest, or struggle to stand up, stop the test and make a note of the repetitions completed.
5. Repeat until you are unable to complete further repetitions, then make a note of your total repetitions completed.

Compare your results to the norms on the table on the next page for body-weight squats.[17]

Ratings for women (squat test) based on age

Age	18–25	26–35	36–45	46–55	56–65	65+
Excellent	>43	>39	>33	>27	>24	>23
Good	37–43	33–39	27–33	22–27	18–24	17–23
Above average	33–36	29–32	23–26	18–21	13–17	14–16
Average	29–32	25–28	19 –22	14–17	10–12	11–13
Below average	25–28	21–24	15–18	10–13	7–9	5–10
Poor	18–24	13–20	7–14	5–9	3–6	2–4
Very poor	<18	<13	<7	<5	<3	<2

Push-up test

The push-up test can evaluate muscular strength and endurance in the upper body – the chest, shoulders and triceps.

Medical and sports research has historically focused on the male body, and this lack of female-specific data means that guidelines and recommendations rely on data gained from studying male subjects. The bias in healthcare is due to several factors, including a desire to protect potential pregnancies from drugs and treatments, research being harder to standardise due to varying hormone levels during a woman's menstrual cycle, and the US Food and Drug Administration recommendation that women should not be included in clinical trials following the thalidomide scandal in 1977. The lack of sports research in women is influenced by similar factors as well as historical biases and assumptions about women's athletic capabilities. Women have only officially been able to enter the Boston Marathon since 1972, before this it was thought that marathon running was too arduous for women. In future, more female-centric sports studies could aid athletic performance, training protocols and approaches to exercise.

The push-up test involves completing as many push ups as possible in 1 minute. As no normative data is available for women completing a full push up, this test requires that women use a modified position (on the knees).

1. To perform the push-up test, start from the top, arms fully extended. Get someone to start a stopwatch.

2. Lower yourself down until your chest is 8cm from the floor, before returning to the start position.
3. You can rest at the top, as necessary, during the test.
4. Complete as many repetitions as possible in 1 minute and take a note of them.

Compare your results to the age-adjusted standards based on guidelines published by the American College of Sports Medicine (ACSM).[18]

Ratings for women (modified push ups) based on age

Age	20–29	30–39	40–49	50–59	60+
Excellent	>48	>39	>34	>29	>19
Good	34–48	25–39	20–34	15–29	5–19
Average	17–33	12–24	8–19	6 –14	3–4
Poor	6–16	4–11	3–7	2–5	1–2
Very Poor	<6	<4	<3	<2	<1

As there is no normative data for women completing a full push up, I have also included the ratings for men based on age. If you are able to complete full push ups you may want to compare your results to this instead.

Ratings for men (full push ups) based on age

Age	20–29	30–39	40–49	50–59	60+
Excellent	>54	>44	>39	>34	>29
Good	45–54	35–44	30–39	25–34	20–29
Average	35–44	24–34	20–29	15–24	10–19
Poor	20–34	15–24	12–19	8–14	5–9
Very Poor	<20	<15	<12	<8	<5

Measuring balance

Several factors influence your ability to balance. The vestibular system, inside the inner ear, is part of the sensory system that informs the brain about balance and motion. The brain then processes this information and sends signals to the rest of the body to maintain balance. Consequently, inner ear issues can lead to problems with balance. As we get older the vestibular system can be slower to react to movement, and this is one reason why the ability to balance can decrease with age.[19]

But loss of balance, or an inability to find balance, can also be a result of a lack of muscular strength and endurance, weak abdominal muscles, visual impairment, poor circulation, a change in blood pressure, some medications, low blood sugar and some neurological conditions.

Single leg balance test

This is a simple balance test with no norm tables to compare to. But one study has found an inability to stand on one foot for 10 seconds, in adults over 50, is associated with a higher risk of death from all causes within the next decade.

This test allows you to benchmark your current ability to balance and provides something against which you can gauge progress on subsequent testing.

1. To perform the test, stand barefoot with feet hip distance apart.
2. When you are ready, lift one foot off the ground and start a timer. The test is over when your foot touches the ground, you hop or you lose balance.
3. Make a note of the time, then repeat with the other leg.
4. You may want to record the best of three attempts.

To increase difficulty, you could rise up onto your toes or close your eyes while performing the test.[20]

The sock and shoe test (also referred to as the 'old person's test')

This is a test of balance, flexibility and strength. There are no standards or norm tables for this test, but it's a fun challenge that you may enjoy trying.

You need a pair of shoes with laces (trainers are ideal) and a pair of ankle socks for this test.

1. Place the trainers and socks on the floor. Put the left trainer on the left-hand side and the right one on the right-hand side, with a sock next to each shoe.
2. Stand barefoot and lift your left foot off the floor.
3. Now reach down, pick up the sock, and put it on your left foot without touching the foot to the floor. Don't cross the leg over the other leg or use it as a support.
4. Once you have put the sock on, reach down whilst keeping the left foot elevated and off the floor, and pick up the left trainer. Now put the trainer on and do up the laces.
5. Now you are ready to change legs.
6. Put the left foot down and at the same time lift the right foot, so that you have hopped from one leg to the other and at no point have both feet on the ground.
7. Repeat the whole process of putting the sock and then the shoe on the right foot.

There are several possible outcomes. You may find this test too difficult and are unable to complete it, you could find you are able to maintain balance long enough to put one sock on but then your balance falters, or you may find you can only complete this test on one side. Whatever the outcome, it can simply be a fun challenge to revisit from time to time and see if there are any changes in your ability to perform it.

You now have a better understanding of what the health- and skills-related components of fitness are. The active-agers exercise recommendations will be based on addressing these components, to support healthier ageing and promote functional movement for life.

There are clear links between the benefits of physical activity and health. Quantifying the amount and type of activity we should do to support health is important so that we can optimise our time and reduce the risk of injury.

The Chief Medical Officers (CMOs) of England, Scotland, Ireland and Wales have drawn up physical activity guidelines for adults in the

UK. These guidelines include type of exercise, volume, duration and frequency necessary to support health.[21]

The current physical activity guidelines (2019) for adults (19 to 64 years) in the UK are:

- Aim to be physically active every day – doing something is better than nothing.
- Undertake muscle-strengthening activities a minimum of twice weekly.
- Accumulate 150 minutes of moderate cardiovascular activity (like walking or cycling), or 75 minutes of vigorous cardiovascular intensity (like running) each week, or a combination of the two.
- Minimise time spent being sedentary and intersperse periods of inactivity with movement and physical activity.[22]

CHAPTER 2

AN INTRODUCTION TO ACTIVE AGEING

What influences physical fitness?

Globally, over a quarter of the world's population do not engage in enough physical activity to support health, which equates to one in three women and one in four men not meeting the recommended physical activity guidelines.

There are individual, social and environmental factors that can influence your ability to be physically active. Individual barriers to exercise can include lack of time, perception of the skills required, fear of judgement, body image issues, increasing age, as well as health or medical concerns. Social barriers to exercise may include lack of childcare or support from family members, partners and friends. Environmental factors include accessibility of suitable fitness facilities, lack of safe or traffic-free outdoor spaces, availability of public transport and lack of resources or equipment.

The factors that can influence our ability to engage in physical activity are also referred to as barriers. Some are real and will need suitable strategies to overcome. For example, an injury may limit the range of exercises that are safe to do, and working around this will require suitable alternatives that don't aggravate the injury. Other barriers may be perceived, such as believing exercise can be dangerous to older adults. This is where education about the benefits of exercise, and support and information about the right type of exercise, is important.

This book aims to address some of these barriers, and the exercises included can be completed in the privacy of your own home with minimal equipment.

Health and physical fitness are also influenced by modifiable and non-modifiable factors. Modifiable factors are things we can influence. So, for example, a sedentary lifestyle is a risk to health, but reducing time spent being sedentary and engaging in regular activity lowers this risk. Modifiable factors include smoking, diet quality, body mass index, physical activity and alcohol intake. Addressing these modifiable factors will help reduce the risk of developing health issues such as cardiovascular disease, type 2 diabetes, strokes, high blood pressure and some cancers. Non-modifiable factors include increasing age, genetics, family history, race/ethnicity and gender. (A gender health gap between men and women exists globally, with men at greater risk of adverse health outcomes than women. However, in the UK this is reversed, and women experience poorer health outcomes than men. For example, studies have shown that women with dementia are monitored less frequently than men by health professionals and have an increased likelihood of being prescribed potentially harmful medication. Common mental health conditions also affect more women than men in the UK, and less is known about female specific health conditions such as endometriosis, which can lead to a delay in diagnosis and treatment.[1, 2])

Although we can't do anything about these non-modifiable risk factors, physical activity will still help support your health.

As you grow older you are at an increased risk of developing some diseases and medical conditions, such as osteoarthritis. But exercise may still be beneficial in slowing down the progression of disease, promoting function and your ability to enjoy and engage in the activities of daily life.

The ageing process

Throughout your lifespan every cell in your body changes. Senescence is the process of growing old at a cellular level, where cells work less efficiently, stop dividing, then die off. Tissues shrink, organs don't work as efficiently, the body breaks down and is unable to function properly, which ultimately leads to death.

Ageing is a lifelong biological process. It starts from birth and encompasses the development of a baby into a child, then young adult, through adulthood, middle age, older age and ultimately the end of life. Many people don't appreciate that ageing is the process of growing up as well as growing old, whereas the deterioration that most people think of as 'ageing' is cell senescence.

You may associate older age with frailty, osteoporosis, heart disease and dementia. Although these are common, they should not be confused with the normal process of ageing, but instead be recognised as indicators of accelerated ageing.[3]

Types of ageing

Ageing means different things to different people. 'You're as young as you feel' and 'Age is just a number' are phrases people commonly use when referring to age. But age, and how we age, is complex and cannot be summarised like this. There is huge diversity in ageing, as evidenced by some 90-year-olds who run marathons while others are physically frail and unable to care for themselves.

Whilst ageing is defined as the process of growing older, we can differentiate further by the type of ageing.

Chronological ageing

Chronological ageing refers to the time that has elapsed since your birth, and it is measured in years, months, weeks, days and seconds.

Chronological ageing applies linearly and consistently to everyone.

Biological ageing

Biological ageing (also known as physiological or functional ageing) refers to the changes and damage to cells, organs and tissues in the body that accumulate with age. These lead to physical signs of ageing, including joint diseases like osteoarthritis, frailty, hearing loss and changes in eyesight. Some of these physiological changes are partly linked to chronological age, but they do not happen linearly or consistently to everyone. The impact of biological ageing explains in part why some 90-year-olds are able to live independently whilst others need help with basic functions of daily life.

Psychological ageing

Psychological ageing refers to how old you feel and may influence how you behave and act regardless of your chronological age. This concept of ageing, as it applies to you, includes subjective age, age identity, attitudes towards ageing, perception of age and satisfaction with age.[4]

Studies into psychological ageing suggest there is a relationship between age identity (how old you feel) and health, cognitive function, wellbeing and longevity.[5]

This concept of psychological ageing helps explain why some people in their eighties assert they feel young (and enjoy a full and active life), whereas other people say they feel old in their fifties and sixties (and act accordingly).

Social ageing

Social ageing refers to how a person's roles, responsibilities and relationships change over time. This includes the roles, responsibilities and relationships with family members, as well as friendships. These changes also apply to the workplace, organisations and wider community.

How ageing is perceived, and the assumptions and expectations from wider society, also impacts social ageing. This can differ according to where we live and the communities that we are part of.

Societal expectations of ageing include how we should behave and what we should like, or be doing, according to our age. In societies that have a positive outlook on ageing this can influence the individual's experience of ageing. Likewise, in societies where ageing is perceived as negative, an individual's experience of ageing is reflective of this.

Social ageing can impact our experience of ageing, in both a positive and negative way depending on how we and society perceive ageing and the assumptions that are made.[6, 7]

Growing older

We can't influence chronological age, which happens consistently and linearly to everyone, but we don't have to be a passive observer of biological, psychological and social ageing. Instead, with an active-ageing approach, we can aim to positively influence all three.

Ageing trajectory

Many people imagine we remain at a constant level throughout our adult lives and decline at some point during our seventies or eighties. The truth is, we are actually in a state of physical decline from our twenties and thirties onwards.[8]

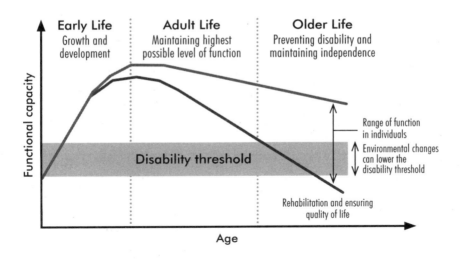

How we age, from a functional perspective, broadly falls into three categories:

1. Optimal ageing: Retaining the highest possible level of
   functional capacity, preventing disability and maintaining
   independence.
2. Normal ageing: Slow and gradual decline in body function, but
   an absence of disease.
3. Accelerated ageing: Rapid deterioration in functional capacity,
   crossing the disability threshold, loss of independence and
   needing assistance for living.

These ageing trajectories, and rate of decline, can be influenced
both positively and negatively through lifestyle behaviours.

Factors such as poor diet, sedentary lifestyle, smoking and stress
have a detrimental effect on health and can increase the average rate
of decline, leading to accelerated ageing. Whereas a healthy diet, an
active lifestyle and good stress-management strategies can help slow
down the rate of physical decline, promoting optimal ageing.

Active ageing plays an important role in both health span and
lifespan. It's helpful to clarify some commonly used terms here.

- Lifespan refers to the number of years a person is alive for.
- Life expectancy refers to the average number of years a person
  can expect to live for.
- Health span refers to the number of years during which a
  person experiences reasonably good health.
- Healthy life expectancy refers to the number of years during
  which a person can expect to live in reasonably good health.

Lifespan and life expectancy are easier to quantify than health
span and healthy life expectancy.

When someone dies their lifespan can be clearly defined as the
number of years, months, days and weeks they were alive for. Average
life expectancy is influenced by several factors, and differs around
the world, but life expectancy at birth in the UK between 2020 and
2022 was 78.6 for men and 82.6 for women.

Health span is subjective and harder to quantify, as it is based on
how an individual perceives their general health and the number of
years reported as 'very good' or 'good health'. Likewise, the data on

healthy life expectancy is based on gathering self-rated assessments from thousands of people, to estimate 'average' healthy life expectancy.

Healthy life expectancy in the UK between 2018 and 2020 was 62.8 for men and 63.6 for women. These statistics reveal the gap between life expectancy and healthy life expectancy, which is between 17 to 20 years for men and women. These represent the number of years men and women in the UK can expect to spend in poorer states of health.

These are the years we are seeking to address as an active ager; to increase the number of years spent in 'good' health and extend healthy life expectancy. The lifestyle factors that increase healthy life expectancy can also extend life expectancy. But an active-ageing approach is primarily focused on improving our quality of life as we grow older, not merely extending life.

Healthy life expectancy is also referred to as 'disability-free' years or Disability-Free Life Expectancy (DFLE). This is an estimate of the average number of years lived without restrictions to activity, due to a physical or mental health condition. Years with disability – the gap – are the years lived with activity restrictions.[9, 10]

In normal human development, from birth through childhood, functional ability increases. Babies and young children require their basic needs to be met by others, which include being fed, cleaned and kept safe from harm, as well as attention to their emotional wellbeing and development. When we are very young our survival depends on these things.

By the time we reach adulthood, and excluding a limiting disability, we can meet our own needs and function independently. Our functional independence as an adult enables us to take care of our basic needs without the assistance of others. These functions, which are essential for living independently, are often referred to as Activities of Daily Living (ADLs) and Instrumental Activities of Daily Living (IADLs).

Babies and young children learn to master some of the essential ADLs as they develop. ADLs include basic tasks that keep you safe, fed, healthy and clean – such as getting dressed and undressed, showering, personal grooming, feeding yourself and walking.

IADLs include tasks that we start to learn as teenagers and young adults. These are often more complex tasks that require cognitive skills of reasoning, judgement and comprehension, and allow us to live independently within society. IADLs include preparing and cooking meals, managing finances, managing means of transportation and travel, managing communications by phone, email and text, maintaining living accommodation and cleaning.[11]

As an active ager our aim is to stay above the disability threshold, maintaining a good level of physical function and independence.

Slowing down the natural rate of decline will impact functional capacity and support the maintenance of ADLs and IADLs. As we have discovered, both ADLs and IADLs are critical for independent living. Of these two the IADLs are often the first tasks that older adults may start to struggle with and find more challenging.

Take a moment now to consider older adults you know, such as your grandparents, parents or those in your community. Have you noticed those who appear to be robust, independent and physically capable in their eighties and older? What about the others, though, the older adults who seem to be struggling a little? Perhaps managing communications is something that's becoming harder for an older adult that you know, or they are finding travelling more challenging. Preparing and cooking meals, maintaining living accommodation and cleaning are other tasks that may become harder. The loss of these IADLs can impact quality of life for some older adults, but with the right support many will still be able to lead a reasonably independent life. You may be in a position of supporting an older relative or neighbour with some of these tasks and are aware of the difference your help makes to their quality of life.

The loss of ADLs, and an inability to take care of basic needs like getting dressed and undressed, using the toilet, showering and feeding yourself, has more serious consequences though. Ultimately, this leads to a requirement of full-time care.

Many people think of ageing as a collection of diseases and impairments, such as frailty, heart disease, strokes and dementia. But these are all disorders of the human body, and although incredibly common should not be viewed as part of the normal ageing process. Genetics do play a part in some disease development, but our own actions have a significant impact on ageing trajectory. Some of the diseases we typically associate with growing older are diseases of inactivity, the result of a sedentary lifestyle, a poor diet and nutrient deficiency.

However, it's important to acknowledge the social, cultural and economic factors that impact disease development but are outside individual control. These factors can all influence dietary quality, choices and availability, exercise and sports, opportunities to be physically active, and lifestyle. Where you live can make a significant difference to your life expectancy. For example, in the UK, life expectancy for women in Kensington and Chelsea is set at 88 years, whereas in Glasgow City it is 78 years.[12]

Influencing your ageing trajectory

Now we've examined the ageing process, we can start to consider ways to reduce the risk of accelerated ageing and to promote healthier ageing.

This is where the components of fitness are relevant. By addressing each component we can influence functional capacity and ability, reduce the risks of developing some diseases and extend healthy life expectancy.

For many of us this won't mean the absence of disease, disability or a challenging medical condition. I have osteoarthritis, have had three shoulder surgeries, and I am typing this whilst recovering from fracturing my wrist after an unfortunate accident. Influencing your ageing trajectory means supporting the healthiest version of you and working around challenges like these.

Supporting body composition

Body composition (bone, muscle and fat) can change during lifespan (see page 3). A loss or gain in body weight is determined by something known as energy balance. Energy is measured in calories, and comes from the food and drink you consume. Energy expenditure is made up of the energy required to maintain basic and life-sustaining functions known as your basal metabolic rate (BMR), the thermic effect of food consumed (TEF) and all physical activity.

When energy intake equals energy expenditure, body weight remains stable. When energy intake exceeds energy expenditure, body weight increases. Likewise, when energy intake is lower than energy expenditure, body weight decreases.

Body composition is an important factor in supporting health and longevity. Maintaining the retention of lean muscle is critical to functional ability as we grow older. Our bodies become less able to respond to dietary protein intake as we age; referred to as blunted muscle protein synthesis and anabolic resistance. This is where strength training alongside the consumption of adequate levels of protein for active agers is vital.

Hormonal changes during menopause impact fat storage, increasing the likelihood of excess body fat being stored centrally in the body as visceral fat. Where we store excess fat is significant. Prior to menopause, women tend to store excess fat in the hips and thighs, which has less associated health risks. Whereas an excess of body fat, in particular visceral fat in the abdomen and surrounding vital organs, is associated with numerous risks to health.

A combination of diet and exercise play an important role in the retention of lean muscle and slowing down the associated muscle loss from blunted muscle protein synthesis.[13]

Low muscle mass and higher body fat levels are associated with poorer health outcomes. Likewise, low body fat levels and excessive leanness are also detrimental to health. Getting this balance right as we grow older can become challenging.

Alongside increasing levels of obesity worldwide, another scenario is receiving greater recognition – sarcopenic obesity. Sarcopenic obesity describes the condition of declining muscle mass and function, combined with increased levels of body fat. This has significant consequences on health such as an increased risk of frailty, falls, disability and a decrease in lifespan.

The proportion of bone in relation to fat and muscle is also an important constituent of body composition. Adults reach peak bone mineral density (BMD) is their twenties, at which point it starts to decline again. The amount of bone loss post-menopause is a subject of debate. Some research has concluded that BMD loss increases substantially in perimenopause and early post-menopause years.[14]

More recently, research has shown that bone loss after menopause is significantly lower than previously thought, decreasing by 10 per cent over 25 years post-menopause. As women now live, on average, a third of their lives post-menopause, further long-term research is needed in this area.[15]

Regardless of the precise percentage of bone loss post-menopause, any reduction in BMD from the peak achieved in your twenties poses a potential risk to health span and lifespan.

Better bone health can be supported through a combination of diet and exercise, in particular resistance and weight-bearing exercises.

Keep in mind that body weight alone does not indicate health status. It should never be assumed that someone in a larger body is 'unhealthy', or someone in a leaner body is 'healthy'. Health and physical fitness are multifactorial. Having an awareness of body composition rather than body weight may be more helpful as an active ager, along with the lifestyle factors that support the retention of lean muscle and reduce the loss of bone mineral density.

Supporting cardiovascular fitness

Our ability to utilise oxygen, critical to the respiratory system that's involved with breathing, decreases with age. Cardiovascular fitness is measured as VO_2 max, as we discovered on page 19. There is a strong correlation between higher VO_2 max scores and longevity, which highlights the importance of cardiovascular fitness in an active-ageing strategy.[16]

From the age of 30 onwards, VO_2 max decreases with age at a rate of about 10 per cent per decade. Although VO_2 max is affected by age, you can slow down this rate of decline with regular cardiovascular exercise. This is especially important if your VO_2 max is on the fair– poor end of the spectrum, as a VO_2 max score > 17.5 ml/kg/min is necessary for an independent lifestyle.

Cardiovascular exercise plays an important role in active ageing to support heart health, reduce the risk of cardiovascular diseases and enjoy everyday activities, like walking, without getting breathless.

Supporting flexibility

Many factors influence flexibility; the ability of muscles, joints and soft tissues to move through an unrestricted, pain-free range of motion. These factors include lifestyle, lack of activity, joint structure, injury, age and gender (women tend to be more flexible than men).

Some people are naturally more flexible with little to no effort, and as many as one in four people are thought to have hypermobility. Hypermobility is where you are able to move some or all of your joints through a greater range of movement than would be considered a 'normal' range. This can sometimes be seen as an advantage in sports and activities like dancing and yoga, but hypermobility can also cause painful joints and other associated problems.

However you view your current level of flexibility, having an adequate range of flexibility is beneficial at every age. Flexibility supports freedom of movement, as well as promoting better posture, reducing joint restrictions and muscle tightness and soreness. Flexibility and stretching also promote relaxation, decreasing tension in the body.

Most of us will lose some degree of flexibility with age. This is partly due to age-related structural changes. Collagen is an important protein found throughout the body, present in bones, muscles, tendons and cartilage. But as collagen naturally decreases with age, this in turn influences flexibility. The amount of lubrication in a joint, and cartilage breakdown – seen in osteoarthritis – can also influence a pain-free range of movement.

Attempting to quantify the exact loss of flexibility associated with age, one study of men and women between the ages of 55–86 years found a decrease in shoulder and hip flexibility of six degrees per decade, with significant decreases observed over the age of 70.[17]

Aside from increasing age, lack of activity is another important factor that influences flexibility. If you are not putting your joints and muscles through their full range of movement on a regular basis, then you'll start to lose the end ranges of these movements.

Flexibility training is an important element of active ageing. Through making stretching part of your regular routine, you'll be able to support the retention of pain-free range of movement in your joints and promote better physical function with age.

Supporting muscular strength and endurance

The growth and maintenance of skeletal muscle relies on physical activity and adequate protein intake. Muscular strength and endurance require the retention of lean muscle. However, muscle strength, alongside muscle size and power, decreases with age. This is also combined with a loss of muscle fibre, especially fast-twitch muscle fibres responsible for fast and explosive movement. The rate of decline can be anywhere between 3 and 8 per cent every decade after the age of 30.

These age-related changes can be offset with strength training, which not only supports the retention of lean muscle but also aids functional ability and quality of life as you grow older.

Strength training is a key strategy in your active-ageing toolbox.

Supporting skill-related components of fitness

The skill-related components of fitness, agility, balance, coordination, power, reaction time and speed are closely related. A loss of one often impacts the others.

A decline in these skills is often associated with age. Some of this can be attributed to a lack of activity that promotes the retention of these skills, but a decrease in any of the health-related components of fitness will also impact these skill-based components.

Agility, balance, coordination, power, reaction time and speed are often evident in older adults who enjoy sports like badminton, walking football and dance. But even if you don't enjoy sporting activities, retention of the skill-related components of fitness can help support healthier ageing.

Including some specific exercises to target these skill-based activities will form part of our active-ageing approach.

Ageism

'Everybody wants to live forever, but nobody wants to be old.'

Jonathan Swift

How do you feel about age? Does growing older fill you with dread? Have you watched relatives or friends struggle with health issues as they have grown older? Do you believe 'good' or 'bad' genetics determines how you will age?

Many things influence our attitude to age and growing older. Societal expectations, family and friends, the communities you are part of, your physical appearance and your health all play a role in how you feel about ageing.

You may have very negative feelings about growing older and believe this will be a time of diminishing function, beset with health issues, loneliness and isolation. You may equate older with unattractiveness, being boring, out of touch and getting slower.

Perhaps you have a more optimistic view on growing older, and see this as an age of opportunity, with greater leisure time, more financial freedom or the joy of being a grandparent. Acknowledging your feelings on ageing are important and relevant to your active-ageing journey.

Dr Charlotte Ord, Counselling Psychologist and author of *Body Confident You: Body Confident Kid,* shares her thoughts on exploring feelings on growing older and ageing.

'It's useful to be curious about what has influenced your feelings about growing older and contributed to your negative perspective. What were your parents' views on getting older? What messages about ageing are being conveyed in your online and offline environments? Who are you following on social media and how is ageing being represented?'

Tackling the negative narrative on ageing is something I have been addressing via my social media accounts for many years. I don't subscribe to the idea that women have a 'best-before' date, or that we need to try to appear youthful to have worth. Instead, I think it helps to define what's important to us as we grow older.

Dr Ord explains how being clear on your values can be a useful guide for behaviour.

'Once you're clear on what matters most to you it's helpful to think about how these fit with ageing. For example, someone with difficult thoughts about her body might avoid going swimming with her grandchildren, which moves her away from her value of being a fun-loving and active grandparent.'

Many of us probably have mixed emotions about growing older and recognise there are some positives and some negatives. Being an active ager isn't about denying some of the aspects about growing older that we find challenging. Instead, it means taking action to support the healthiest version of ourselves, and making peace with some of the aspects of ageing that we may struggle with. An approach Dr Ord also endorses.

'Moving towards a place of acceptance with your body and the ageing process is really about building your tolerance for uncomfortable thoughts and feelings and choosing to act in line with your values regardless.'

The World Health Organization (WHO) defines ageism as 'the stereotypes (how we think), prejudice (how we feel) and discrimination (how we act) towards others or oneself based on age'.[18]

Ageism has a huge influence on us as individuals, as a wider society and the economy. To embrace active ageing we need to confront the influence that ageism has on us. This can be both challenging and uncomfortable. We might not want to acknowledge all the ways in which we are ageist, or have been in the past, to ourselves and others in our thoughts, words and actions.

Ageism can affect people of all ages. In Europe, for example, younger people report more perceived ageism than other age groups. But in the context of active ageing, we are primarily concerned with ageism as it relates to growing older. This is a significant global issue, with one in two people said to be ageist against older people.

It's not always straightforward to recognise ageism because it's so widespread and effectively normalised. How many of these do you recognise?

'I'm too old to wear this dress.'
'She looks good for her age.'
'Mutton dressed as lamb.'
'I'm having a senior moment.'
'She's ageing like fine wine.'
'Old women are so sweet.'
'People should age gracefully.'
'You can't teach an old dog new tricks.'

There are three types of ageism: institutional ageism, interpersonal ageism and self-directed ageism.

Institutional ageism – this is where institutions perpetuate ageism through rules, practices and policies that discriminate against older adults. It can also be a problem in healthcare settings where older adults are not offered the same treatment options as younger adults. For example: Applicants under 40 encouraged to apply for this exciting opportunity.

Interpersonal ageism – this happens between the interactions of individuals, where one person makes assumptions or jokes or has a dismissive attitude to another based on their age. For example: There's no point applying; you probably won't understand the technology at your age.

Self-directed ageism – this is when an individual internalises ageism. This is normally a result of absorbing ageist messages from society, on how to think, act and behave at certain ages. Internalised ageism then influences thoughts and behaviour. For example: I shouldn't apply, I'm probably too old to learn their IT systems.

Ageism can influence how you feel about exercise, activity, your health and your body.[19]

When negative age stereotypes are portrayed in the media you may believe older adults are an acceptable target for jokes, will usually be in poor health, or are miserable. If you don't see positive examples of active older adults, but instead see athletic younger people exercising, you may believe you are too old to join a gym. If you think older bodies, loose skin and stretch marks are ugly, this can make you feel embarrassed about your own body. In short, you are less likely to take action to support healthier ageing when you believe poor health is inevitable, and older means being less able and undesirable. One study has even demonstrated that how you feel about ageing has an impact on lifespan: individuals with a positive self-perception of ageing live longer on average by 7.5 years than those with a less-positive attitude to ageing.[20]

I can pinpoint the exact moment I suddenly felt 'old' and stereotyped based purely on my age. It was when I was pregnant with my fifth baby at the age of 39. My medical notes referred to me as an elderly multigravida. Elderly in medical terms refers to pregnant women over 35, and multigravida means when it's not your first pregnancy. I was horrified, elderly at the age of 39?! Thankfully this term is no longer used in the UK.

During my forties I had a growing awareness that my age was becoming an issue, something I felt increasingly judged or stereotyped by. I recall working on a stand at a fitness event. A man who was probably in his late twenties came over to ask me about some of the products on the stand, and we got onto the topic of music. I made a mistake and referred to the band 'Two Door Cinema Club' as three instead of two. When I quickly corrected myself, he smirked and said, 'You got it wrong because you're old'. This is a classic example of interpersonal ageism; passing off an ageist statement as a joke.

But nothing could have prepared me for the explosion of ageism I experienced online in October 2021, when I was 58 years old.

I shared a dance video on Instagram that quickly amassed over 11 million views. In my video caption I talked about the benefits of exercise for healthier ageing. And whilst thousands of people appreciated my active-ageing tips, lots of people took issue with my outfit – a checked shirt, a pair of shorts and cowboy boots. The ageist comments were directed at my outfit, dressing like a teenager was the common complaint, and the fact I was dancing – embarrassing for a woman your age to dance on social media – was another one. As someone who wears shorts regularly for exercise and has always loved dancing, I couldn't understand what the fuss was about! Since then, I've experienced online ageism thousands of times. I've been told I'd look younger if I coloured my grey hair, I should be careful I don't break a hip dancing, and I have been referred to as 'granny' more times than I can remember.

With these examples of interpersonal ageism, it's easy to see how this has the potential to influence self-directed ageism. It highlights how prevalent and insidious ageism is.

As an active ager I urge you to challenge your own internalised ageism and increase your awareness of the role ageism plays in society. Addressing ageism not only benefits your physical health and psychological wellbeing, but it can also have a positive influence on the communities and institutions you are part of and has the potential to extend your lifespan.

You don't have to dance on social media or wear shorts, instead try answering the question – what do you think you are too old for? By giving this some thought you may start to identify your own internalised ageism and recognise any self-imposed restrictions.

Longevity – good genetics or just luck?

If you come from a family of centenarians, you might feel your genetics are on your side. If, on the other hand, you have a family history of heart disease, dementia or breast cancer, you may have some valid concerns about your genetic inheritance.

Genetics plays a role in longevity, but it's not as big an influence as some people imagine. It has been estimated that genetic factors account for 25 per cent of the variation of human longevity. The remaining 75 per cent is down to lifestyle, not luck.[21]

The bottom line is you can negatively influence 'good' genetics with poor lifestyle choices, likewise, you can positively influence 'bad' genetics with beneficial lifestyle choices.

To commit to an active-ageing approach, it's important to manage our expectations and recognise any limitations, but ultimately to understand the role we can play in our own ageing trajectory.

Physical activity and exercise can't solve everything, but they can help reduce some of the health risks encountered with increasing age and support healthier ageing – at least, the healthiest version of ourselves, which will be different for everyone.

CHAPTER 3

CHALLENGING CHANGES

'There is no situation, there is no age and no condition where exercise is not a good thing.'

Chief Medical Officer Chris Whitty, 2020[1]

As we grow older, maintaining our health can start to feel like a game of dodgeball. Increasing age is one of those 'non-modifiable risk factors' for cardiovascular disease and a range of other diseases and conditions. Health screening programmes are targeted at those people who may be at an increased risk of certain conditions. Screening aims to offer early detection, intervention and improved outcomes. Typical screening programmes target women during pregnancy and newborn babies, and throughout female lifespan for conditions including breast cancer, cervical cancer, bowel cancer, diabetic retinopathy and other eye examinations.

Health screening provides one way of managing risks, by offering early detection and treatment and increasing the odds in our favour – it's like an extra pair of eyes in a game of dodgeball. Reducing risks to health requires a combination of screening to identify potential risks alongside taking action (like being physically active and eating a healthy diet) to minimise these risks.

There are no guarantees that being physically active will prevent the development of a disease or a life-limiting condition. But it's the most effective way to reduce risks to health, especially as we know physical activity can help prevent and manage over twenty chronic conditions and diseases, including some cancers, heart disease, type 2 diabetes and depression.[2]

However, one in three women worldwide do not do enough physical activity to support their health, and in the UK this figure is even worse, with only one in two women sufficiently active for their health. It is estimated that physical activity can reduce two of the biggest risks to women's health as we grow older – dementia and cardiovascular disease. Women who meet the UK CMOs' guidelines for physical activity stand to reduce the risk of dementia by up to 30 per cent, cardiovascular disease by up to 35 per cent, breast cancer by 20 per cent and hip fractures up to 68 per cent.[3, 4]

You may have a skewed perspective on what's realistic and achievable, though. We can't fail to be influenced by the prevalence of disease in our friends, family and communities.

Talk of reducing our risk to disease can feel challenging, infuriating and sometimes insensitive. Like me, you probably know people who have done everything 'right' and yet have still developed a disease or illness. Not to mention the unpredictability of life, and how everything can change in a heartbeat by simply being in the wrong place at the wrong time, or an accident.

Like my brother who died at the age of 18 years old in a freak accident.

I have witnessed the passing of clients and friends from cancer and other illnesses, women who were active and fit their entire adult lives, and yet they still died too soon and too young.

Mary is one of those women. I first met fellow fitness professional Mary Huckle in 2016 when we shared the stage presenting together at an industry event. Mary spoke movingly about her journey with breast cancer, and the importance and role of physical activity for women during and after treatment.

Mary initially trained as an exercise to music teacher and a personal trainer. She also coached her own running club three times a week and loved the camaraderie she created with her clients. Mary went on to specialise in Pilates instruction as a result of her initial breast cancer diagnosis in 2007. Despite Mary's personal health challenges, she continued to coach and support dozens of women with breast cancer, helping them regain their ability to exercise, with confidence. In July 2014 Mary was diagnosed with secondary cancer during a routine appointment with her oncologist. She became a fierce campaigner for METUPUK, the only secondary breast cancer patient advocacy group in the UK and worked tirelessly to highlight the need for improved funding, education and research.[5]

Sadly, Mary died at the age of 57, peacefully in a hospice in June 2023, surrounded by those she loved.

My own father, who is 87 years old at the time of writing, has recently been diagnosed with prostate cancer. He has been physically active throughout his life. In his younger years he would regularly cycle from Bognor Regis to Southampton and back in a day for 'fun' – a round trip of 80 miles. And in his retirement he has continued to swim several times a week, play golf weekly, spend many hours outdoors gardening and is always up a ladder 'fixing' something or making something.

Reducing risk is not the same as eliminating risk. Unfortunately, it is not possible to eliminate risk; we must make peace with what we can't control, we must accept that life oftentimes feels unfair and we must acknowledge the seeming randomness of catastrophic accidents. Reducing your individual risk is about taking action to stack the odds in your favour for your current and future health. An active-ageing approach is the best defence you have in your armoury against chronic disease.

Noncommunicable diseases (NCDs), also known as chronic diseases, are the leading cause of death worldwide. Chronic diseases include cardiovascular diseases, respiratory diseases, diabetes, obesity, cancers and strokes. The proportion of deaths arising due to chronic diseases worldwide is increasing; in 1990, 57 per cent of deaths worldwide were attributed to a chronic disease, by 2016 this figure had increased to 72 per cent. Current trends and estimates suggest life expectancy will be reduced for future generations due to this upward trajectory in chronic diseases.

This worldwide growth in deaths from chronic disease can be attributed to a combination of genetic, physiological, environmental and behavioural factors. As active agers we are once again faced with addressing what we can control, alongside recognising the things that are out of our individual control – like genetic factors and air pollution.

The risk of developing a chronic disease increases in people who smoke, are physically inactive, eat an unhealthy diet and consume too much alcohol. The metabolic changes that are a warning indicator to chronic disease development include raised blood pressure, obesity, hyperglycaemia (high blood glucose levels) and hyperlipidaemia (high levels of fat in the blood).

Whilst the evidence that physical activity supports healthier ageing is overwhelming, we can often face challenges and barriers (perceived and real) to being more active as we grow older.

Physical challenges can include joint pain or restriction, pelvic floor weakness, balance problems, previous injury, fatigue, an existing medical condition and the side effects of medications. But almost every physical challenge you face can be overcome by adapting and modifying exercise to your specific needs. So, for women with pelvic floor weakness, we can exclude exercises that are likely to increase downward pressure on the pelvic floor and lead to stress incontinence. For anyone with a reduced range of movement in the shoulder joint we exclude exercises that can increase the likelihood of shoulder impingement, alongside including exercises that promote mobility and stabilisation. As CMO Chris Whitty says, 'There is no situation, there is no age and no condition where exercise is not a good thing.'

It can be frustrating accepting some of these physical changes and challenges that we face. If I dwell too long on what I used to be able to do, before I had three shoulder surgeries and developed osteoarthritis, I feel despondent and disappointed. Coming to terms with these changes requires a certain amount of letting go, much like the process of grieving, until we can reach a place of acceptance and find a new way of going forward. This often necessitates adapting when it comes to exercise. Playing the long game means training smarter not harder, doing enough exercise to support healthier ageing and modifying as necessary to stay the right side of injury and reduce the risk of further surgery.

Making peace with a health issue as we grow older can be very challenging. Dr Charlotte Ord offers her thoughts on this.

'Having worked in NHS pain management services I understand how facing a physical health challenge can feel defeating and often hopeless. It's confronting not only in the sense of sometimes having to redefine

your identity and purpose, but also means that we must (at least to some extent) face our own fallibility and mortality. I think this can be a positive thing, however. It reminds us that we all have a deadline and that we don't have infinite time in this life. It's about what we want to do with our time.'

Exercise prescription is about making sure exercise is safe and effective. The success of a session is not measured in how sweaty you get, or how sore you are afterwards. As an active ager the focus is on safety first, avoiding injury that could impact your training for months, and exercise that doesn't leave you feeling depleted and unable to move for a week, and instead leaves you feeling energised.

This doesn't mean an end to new training goals or competitive pursuits, though. Plenty of people continue to run marathons and take part in various other fitness events, like the CrossFit Games and Hyrox, in their forties, fifties and older. In recent years there's been wider recognition that older athletes need their own divisions when competing in these events, especially when you take into consideration the average age of a CrossFit games competitor – 29 years old in 2023. In 2010 CrossFit introduced a masters division for athletes over 50, adding further age divisions each year. In 2021 CrossFit introduced two new age divisions – men and women aged 60–64, and men and women aged 65+, bringing the total to seven age divisions for master athletes to 35–39, 40–44, 45–49, 50–54, 55–59, 60–64 and 65+. This demonstrates the growing appetite of older adults to test their physical fitness and capabilities against others of a similar age, like Carol Norris.[6]

Carol Norris is a 61-year-old fitness instructor who took part in her first Hyrox competition in 2023. Hyrox is a fitness race that combines running with eight different functional workout stations.

'I have always enjoyed being physically active and going to gyms and taking part in classes like aerobics. But it wasn't until I entered my fifties that I started to lift weights and discovered how much I enjoyed getting stronger.'

Carol had a career working in agriculture, but it was during the Covid pandemic and lockdown that she saw an opportunity to follow her passion and study to become a fitness instructor. 'I've always preferred being on the move, and I had had enough of sitting down, looking at a screen all day.' Carol quickly added to her fitness qualifications, enabling her to teach a range of classes, including Pilates, Barre and Balance.

Functional fitness has always appealed to Carol as well, so when her gym suggested a group of them enter a Hyrox competition she thought it sounded like a great new challenge. 'We didn't really know what we were letting ourselves in for at first.' Nevertheless, Carol enjoyed her first competition and qualified for the World Championships. Several months later, at her second competition, she was delighted when she achieved World Record Holder status in the 60–64 age category.

'My training has evolved over the years. Taking part in Hyrox has added greater variety to my training and made it more focused,' Carol says. 'The functional fitness stations in Hyrox require strength, power and good mobility. There are movement standards you must attain in each exercise for them to count, or you lose marks or get sent back! You need a good level of cardiovascular conditioning as well because there's a lot of running involved between each station. My aim now is to continue to improve my time for the next World Championships!'

Carol is keen to avoid injury, though. 'If anything, I think I am less injury prone now than when I was younger. I teach Pilates several times a week, which involves lots of stretching, and it has made a significant difference to my mobility and flexibility. I am also more focused about my nutrition, and understand how important this is for my training, recovery and performance.'

Carol's advice to other women is simple: 'Don't see yourself as different just because you are older, and don't put a ceiling on what you can achieve!'

Undoubtedly, training for any competitive fitness event is a challenge, and the risk of injury tends to be greater when we are pushing at the limits of our physical capabilities. Older athletes need to be especially mindful of this, being vigilant about exercise preparation through an adequate warm-up, responding quickly to any physical niggles, prioritising sleep and restful recovery and good nutrition.[7]

Sheila Nollert, 67, is another active ager who hasn't let age stop her taking on a challenge. At the age of 65 Sheila embarked on her first solo canoe trip. The location for Sheila's solo adventure was Algonquin Park, in Canada, famous for its wildlife, with over 2,400 lakes.

'The land is rugged, predominantly granite gouged out by glaciers, making for a varied topography of rolling land covered in pines and birch,' Sheila explains.

Sheila's trip lasted four days in total and consisted of paddling a loop of eight lakes for a total of 23km. She had to carry everything she needed for the trip between each lake for 14km before setting up camp each night. This included her food in a bear-proof container, bear spray, cookstove, pot, water purification system, portable transceiver, clothes, sleeping bag, maps and the canoe! 'To portage between each lake, I divided my gear in half, so it was necessary for me to make two trips each time. The first trip always included my 16kg canoe while wearing my small backpack of 5kg. The second trip I carried my larger 14.5kg backpack and my tent which weighed 4.5kg.'

They were long, isolated and tiring days. 'I didn't see a single person from start to finish on my trip. The first and second days I paddled and portaged for five hours to get to the next location to set up my campsite, which took over 45 minutes each time.'

Sheila planned and prepared for months in advance of her solo trip. She knew she had to be ready for both the physical demands it would entail and the practicalities of eating, sleeping and the possibility of crossing paths with a wild bear! 'I planned my route and went over my maps many times. I practised loading my backpack, to fit everything in optimally, and carrying my canoe around the yard. I had to work on my strength, stamina, agility and balance. All skills that were going to be necessary to put in hours of paddling every day, portaging my gear and lifting my canoe overhead.'

Sheila knew it was imperative not to get injured and that she'd face steep hills, embankments, rocks and tree roots as she portaged between each lake. 'I took up meditation as well. Being alone in the wilderness, especially at night in the tent, I thought it would be a good way to calm any racing thoughts I might have.'

Sheila's advice to other women contemplating any sort of adventure or challenge is this. 'It's easy to play safe in our everyday lives. We put off things, and risk never getting round to them. If there's something you've always wanted to do give it some serious consideration. I yearned to do a solo canoe trip for a long time, it would have been a tragedy if I'd kept putting it off. I'm so pleased I finally made it happen. It taught me I can do hard things, and I still feel a tremendous sense of accomplishment that I achieved my dream.'

Not everyone wants to take part in a competitive fitness event like Carol, or a solo canoe trip like Sheila, but perhaps you have concerns about gentler pursuits, and other forms of exercise. If so, you're not alone. Fear of injury can be a barrier to exercise in older adults. The results of one study revealed that as many as 1 in 10 adults over 55 in the UK don't exercise regularly or wouldn't join a gym through fear of getting injured, and half don't think exercise is an important lifestyle choice, or essential to support bone density in older age.[8]

Whilst physical activity is the best way to support your health and preserve your mobility and function, it is important to consider the best ways to minimise risks to important structures like bones, joints, tendons and muscles. Common exercise-induced injuries can include overuse injuries, rotator cuff tears, stress fractures and meniscus tears. Many of these can be avoided through engaging in a variety of different movement patterns, allowing sufficient recovery between sessions and responding to 'niggles' quickly.[9, 10, 11, 12]

CHAPTER 4

UNDERSTANDING MENOPAUSE

It is just over 11 years since I went through menopause.

In the preceding decade my periods had become erratic and unpredictable. In my late thirties I discussed concerns about my cycle with my doctor, who told me, 'You are most likely perimenopausal.' I remember being shocked at the time, because I thought I was too young to be experiencing symptoms that might be linked to menopause.

Despite my erratic cycle, much to my delight I did manage to conceive and give birth to my fifth and final baby at the age of 40. My periods continued to be erratic and unpredictable for the next nine years, though.

I was around 49 years old when I had what I thought was my last period. Eleven months passed by without a period and then – bam! – another period came along just when I thought they were over.

I had a further couple of cycles before my periods ceased again for good. I was 51 at the time, which coincidentally is also the average age of menopause for women in the UK.

It's only with the benefit of hindsight I can appreciate the numerous perimenopause symptoms I experienced during my forties, including hot flushes, heart palpitations, insomnia, brain fog and skin irritation.

In the early 2000s women had little in the way of menopause education, support and advice. Women experiencing perimenopause symptoms and menopause at this time were exposed to confusing information regarding the use of HRT (hormone replacement therapy), despite it being in use and available to women in the UK since 1965.

A high level of media interest followed the publication of the 2002 Women's Health Initiative (WHI) study. The WHI clinical trial started in 1993 to look at the health effects of women taking oestrogen-only

HRT or combined HRT (oestrogen and progesterone), with women taking a placebo. In 2002 the WHI halted the area of the study that was looking at the health effects of combined HRT (oestrogen and progesterone). The study raised safety concerns with the use of combined HRT and found a small increase in risk of breast cancer, heart disease, stroke and blood clots. The health headlines that followed frightened doctors and women alike. Doctors were concerned for their patients, and many stopped prescribing any type of HRT – both the oestrogen-only HRT and the combined HRT. Women already taking HRT were advised to stop taking it. For others, approaching menopause and experiencing perimenopause symptoms for the first time, advice and treatment options became limited as a result.[1]

In 2004 the oestrogen-only arm of the WHI HRT study ended, finding some beneficial effects for breast cancer, and cardiovascular disease risk, and a small increased risk of stroke. But the continued confusion and concerns about associated health risks with HRT meant that by 2007 HRT use fell from two million women to one million women in the UK.

The WHI study is now widely recognised as flawed. One striking problem was the age of the women in the study, only one in six were within five years of menopause, the rest were much older. In the WHI study 33 per cent of the women were aged 50–59 years, 45 per cent were aged 60–69 years and 21 per cent were aged 70–79. Older women are naturally at a greater risk of experiencing some of the health issues identified in the WHI study of combined HRT, including heart disease and stroke.[2]

I was one of those women caught up in the confusion around HRT in the mid-2000s. My knowledge about perimenopause and menopause didn't extend much beyond the most talked-about symptom – hot flushes. Although I had a rudimentary understanding about perimenopause, my doctor did not connect the dots with some of the symptoms I was experiencing, perhaps due to a lack of GP training in menopause at the time. I was unable to make an informed choice about my options, given the continued confusion about the risks and benefits of HRT. In fact, my knee-jerk reaction was – I don't need to take HRT and increase the risk to my health as I led a reasonably healthy lifestyle.

It's only with the benefit of hindsight that I have been able to make sense of my own perimenopause journey in the years between 2005 and 2014.

Perhaps I would have made a different decision and taken HRT with the knowledge I have now.

Over ten years since my last period, insomnia still troubles me. The lifetime risk of insomnia is 40 per cent higher for women than it is for men. Insomnia has troubled me on and off for years and perimenopause triggered more serious bouts of insomnia in me. Fluctuating oestrogen levels often leads to night sweats, hot flushes and frequent trips to the bathroom. Falling levels of oestrogen can also result in extreme skin irritation.

Low levels of progesterone can cause sleep problems, including night sweats, sleep apnea and insomnia. Some studies have shown that HRT can improve sleep quality and may be an effective treatment if other potential causes of insomnia have been eliminated.

It's not widely appreciated that oestrogen plays a significant role in modulating the immune system as well. The immune system consists of cells, organs, tissues and substances that helps the body fight infection and disease, which gradually declines from your thirties onwards.

Dr Jenna Macciochi, immunologist and author of *Immunity: The Science of Staying Well*, explains further.

'This is a process known as immunosenescence, which becomes more pronounced in our fifties and beyond. Menopause marks another critical tipping point due to hormonal changes, particularly the reduction in oestrogen, which has important immunomodulatory effects. These changes in immune function can manifest as tiredness, new diagnoses of autoimmune diseases and poorer responses to infections.'

Lifestyle plays a crucial role in the management of menopause, supporting our immune function and our health post-menopause, which encompasses much of the content of this book. This includes daily movement and physical activity, structured exercise to address the specific health issues associated with menopause, like bone health and cardiovascular health, good nutrition, reducing alcohol intake, stress management strategies and prioritising sleep. If you've successfully addressed all of these lifestyle factors but continue to be troubled by menopause symptoms, what else can you do?

I asked Dr Nighat Arif, a GP who specialises in women's health and author of *The Knowledge: Your Guide to Female Health – From Menstruation to the Menopause*, if it's ever too late to start taking HRT, for women who may feel they have missed out.

> *'Starting systemic HRT, as per NICE guidelines, can be considered at any age for the management of menopausal symptoms. It's never too late to start if you are troubled with symptoms, of which there are 42. Some people will experience mild or no symptoms, others may be troubled by debilitating symptoms. Individual risks versus benefits must be assessed taking into account medical history, family history, personal risk of breast cancer and risk of endometrial hyperplasia. If you do not have any menopausal symptoms, then taking systemic HRT is not recommended or advised by NICE unless considering using systemic HRT for the prevention and treatment of osteoporosis regardless of menopausal symptoms.'* [3]

The menopause movement

In recent years, thanks to the combined efforts of women, doctors with an interest in female health, academics and campaigners, menopause has been in the spotlight and received greater attention. As a result, there is more information, education and advice about menopause now than there was 20 years ago, when I was experiencing my first perimenopause symptoms.

Menopause is no longer the taboo topic it once was in many places around the world. Education, information and support continues to grow. Research and studies on best treatment options are also ongoing. My hope is that my daughters and granddaughters will be better equipped to deal with this life stage when their time comes.

In the meantime, we know a lot about the long-term health implications and how we can support heathier ageing beyond menopause. Let's look at how menopause impacts ageing, and what our active-ageing approach should look like.

Definitions

Before we go any further, let's clarify some definitions:

- Menopause: A year after your last period. The average age for menopause in the UK is 51.
- Premature menopause: When menopause occurs before the age of 40.
- Early menopause: When menopause occurs before the age of 45.
- Perimenopause: The time preceding menopause when a range of symptoms may be experienced. Perimenopause can start anywhere between 8 and 10 years prior to menopause. This means many women will experience symptoms in their early forties.
- Post-menopause: The time when you have not had a period for one year and a day. You will be post-menopause for the rest of your life.

How menopause impacts ageing

As you enter perimenopause and the ovaries start to slow down, the hormones they produce also start to fluctuate. These hormones – oestrogen, progesterone and testosterone – are chemical messengers that travel throughout the body. Although it is widely understood that these hormones are important to the reproductive system, they affect numerous processes throughout the body beyond the reproductive system.

The role of oestrogen in the body
- Brain: Helps regulate mood and body temperature. It also helps with cognition and memory.
- Heart: Has an important function in the heart, as it protects the arteries and lowers blood pressure.
- Bones, muscles and joints: Helps support bone growth and strength and assists joint lubrication. It has an anti-inflammatory effect on joints and muscles as well.

- Pelvic health: Plays an important role in the health of collagen, present in the pelvic floor muscles. It improves bladder function, reduces the risk of infection and aids lubrication.
- Immune function: Has a significant role in immune function, interacting with immune cells, helping maintain immune tolerance and protecting against infections.

The role of progesterone in the body

- Brain: Assists brain cell function, aiding memory, mood and brain Health.
- Bones: Assists bone building.
- Immune function: Helps reduce inflammation and decreases the risk of autoimmune diseases.
- Metabolism: Assists in the regulation of healthy blood sugar levels.
- Psychological wellbeing: Has a sedative effect that helps promote sleep. It also reduces anxiety.
- Muscles: Responsible for stimulating muscle growth.
- Reproduction: Regulates menstruation and supports pregnancy.

The role of testosterone in the body

- Eyes: Reduces dry eyes and assists lubrication.
- Cardiovascular system: Assists the cardiovascular system, helping the efficiency of the heart. It helps blood vessels work better, increasing blood flow.
- Reproductive and sexual function: Important for libido and urogenital health. It can also reduce vaginal dryness and soreness.
- Brain: Aids concentration and memory and contributes to sleep quality.
- Muscles: Assists muscle mass and strength.
- Bones: Increases bone mineral density.
- Pelvic health: Assists bladder function and decreases the risk of infection. It also aids vaginal lubrication, keeping tissues healthy.

Exercise in your peri- to post-menopause years can assist in managing symptoms, improve mood and support your long-term health. And, crucially, exercise helps to counteract the negative impact these hormonal changes have on your heart, muscles, bones and joints, pelvic floor and immune function.

Exercise to support brain health

Dementia has been the UK women's leading cause of death for over a decade. It disproportionally affects women; in 2020, 46,000 women died from dementia compared to 24,000 men. Research in this field is ongoing, and our understanding of the role that menopause has on brain health is still evolving. Science is some way off from providing a cure or treatment to reverse the various forms of dementia. Our best defence, as active agers eager to support our brains and bodies, is to engage in the activities that have been shown to be beneficial to brain health.[4]

Exercise that is fun, engaging, challenging and has a social element to it can be beneficial for brain health, including cognitive function and mood. Cardiovascular exercise is also known to boost blood flow to the brain. The hippocampus is a region of the brain associated with memory, learning and emotions. Hippocampal atrophy refers to brain shrinkage. In one study, older adults who walked for two hours a week were found to be at a decreased risk of hippocampal atrophy, an early characteristic of Alzheimer's disease.[5]

In another study of older adults, one year of aerobic activity was sufficient to enhance hippocampal volume. Improved memory function, through increasing hippocampal volume, was shown to be neuroprotective.[6]

Exercise activities that incorporate cognitive tasks have also been shown to help both maintain and improve cognitive function. Learning a new dance sequence is a great example of aerobic exercise that is also a cognitive challenge. A ball game, which requires predicting and anticipating where the ball will land and responding accordingly, is another great example of a cognitive-challenging exercise.[7]

Exercise to support heart health

Prior to menopause, women have a reduced risk of experiencing a heart attack to men. After menopause, the risk of cardiovascular disease and heart attack increases. Studies have shown how plaque, which increases the risk of heart attacks, starts to build up in women post-menopause. In one such study, post-menopausal women underwent heart scans to assess plaque via a CAC score, which measures fat, calcium and other substances. Each woman in the study was matched to a man of a similar profile to compare CAC scores in men and women. The study showed that women experience a sharp rise in CAC scores post-menopause, indicating a steep build-up of plaque. The rise in CAC scores was lower in men, resulting in a levelling off of cardiovascular disease risk in women post-menopause and an evening up of risks for men and women.[8]

Cardiovascular disease refers to a range of conditions that can affect the heart and blood vessels. These conditions include heart disease – like angina and heart attacks – strokes and vascular dementia.

Oestrogen has a protective effect on your heart, it helps to keep your blood vessels healthy, controls cholesterol levels and reduces the build-up of fatty plaques in your arteries. But although declining oestrogen levels increase cardiovascular disease risk, cardiovascular exercise provides a protective mechanism by which we can support cardiovascular health.[9]

This might be a good time to delve a little deeper into your relationship with cardiovascular exercise, also referred to as aerobic exercise. Cardiovascular exercise has long been promoted as a 'fat-burning' exercise, a means to 'drop a dress size' and make women smaller. This has negatively influenced the way many women feel about cardiovascular exercise. Some women associate 'cardio' with painful, sweaty workouts, coupled with yo-yo, disappointing diets.

If this has been your experience previously, it's important to remember the primary goal of cardiovascular exercise is to support cardiovascular health. This is especially relevant as we grow older. Your heart is the most important muscle in your body, everything relies on it working efficiently. Like other muscles in your body, the heart gets stronger with exercise, increasing in size and pumping blood more effectively. During cardiovascular exercise cardiac output increases, along with blood pressure. You'll be aware of this as your pulse increases, you start to breathe faster than normal and you feel warmer. These are temporary changes, but over time your body adapts to cardiovascular exercise, which leads to a lower resting heart rate and cardiac hypertrophy (increase in size of the heart muscle).

Furthermore, it really doesn't matter what type of cardiovascular activity you do, any activity that increases your heart rate over a sustained period will support heart health.

The additional factor to consider is whether your cardiovascular activity is weight-bearing or non-weight-bearing. Weight-bearing cardiovascular activity, like walking, running or dancing, supports bone health as well as heart health. So, where possible, it's beneficial to include some weight-bearing cardiovascular activities, even if you prefer non-weight-bearing cardiovascular activities like swimming and cycling. It's fine to do these as well, just be aware that strength training is even more important if the only cardio you do is non-weight-bearing.

Exercise to support bones, muscles and joints

Bones are living tissue; they constantly remodel and regenerate throughout our lifetime. The bones in your skeleton have a smooth outer surface and a honeycomb-like mesh structure inside. This honeycomb structure helps contribute to bone strength. When bones weaken, the honeycomb structure starts to break down, leaving the smooth outer layer holding the bone together.

When we are younger, bone remodelling happens at a relatively fast rate; children recover from a broken arm in a matter of weeks in a plaster cast, whereas a hip fracture in our eighties can take many months and poses a significant risk to health and mortality.

Bone mineral density refers to how porous your bones are; peak bone mineral density is reached around the age of 30, after this bone tissue starts to decrease. This is because up until the age of 30 we build more bone than we lose, through the remodelling process.

One year before menopause, and for the following five years, bone mineral density decreases rapidly. The average loss of bone mineral density amounts to a 10 per cent reduction, although some women will lose more.[10]

This loss of bone mineral density increases the risk of developing osteoporosis, making bones weak and vulnerable to breakage. In osteoporosis bones become more porous and brittle as the honeycomb structure starts to break down, creating unsupported patches within the bones.

There is a genetic component to osteoporosis, meaning you are more likely to develop it if you have a family history of this condition.

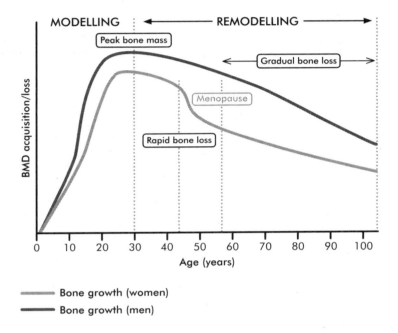

Osteoporosis is a chronic condition that disproportionately affects more women than men. One in three women and one in five men over the age of 50 have osteoporosis, and one in two women over the age of 50 experience a bone fracture as a result. It has been estimated that 200 million people suffer from osteoporosis worldwide, with over 10 million Americans and 3.5 million people in the UK affected.[11]

Although these statistics are grim, you can help slow down this natural decrease in bone mineral density through exercise. The type of exercise you do is significant, though; exercise that supports bone health includes weight-bearing exercise, strength training and exercise that involves impact. This is because bone tissue needs to be exposed to mechanical loading that exceeds that of daily activities.[12]

When you lift weights, for example, forces are exerted on your bones via the muscles pulling on them. Bones are also subject to a force and increased mechanical loading when your foot strikes the ground, and when your hand strikes an object.

Whilst strength training is important for bone health it's also very beneficial in aiding the retention of lean muscle and keeping the supporting structures of joints healthy.

Muscle mass decreases by 3–8 per cent per decade after the age of 30. There is a close link between bone mineral density, lean muscle and exercise. The same exercise approach that supports and slows down the loss of bone mineral density will have a positive impact on the retention of lean muscle.

Joints have numerous oestrogen receptors. Oestrogen plays a protective role in joint health, decreasing inflammation and aiding lubrication. The loss of oestrogen during menopause can lead to joint pain and discomfort in some women. There is also a strong correlation between the onset of perimenopause and joint health issues, such as osteoarthritis. Whilst it may be challenging to exercise when you have achy joints, it's beneficial and important to maintain movement and function in the joints through regular exercise. Strengthening the structures that support a joint, through exercise, can also assist with pain management.

Exercise to support the pelvic floor

The pelvic floor tissues of the vagina, vulva, bladder and bowel have many oestrogen receptors, and, as oestrogen declines throughout the body during menopause, this impacts the pelvic floor. As a result, bladder or bowel symptoms may be experienced, or an existing issue can worsen. This is also a time when a bladder or bowel prolapse can develop.

The loss of skeletal muscle we experience with age also affects the muscles of the pelvic floor. Genitourinary symptoms of menopause (GSM) are also common, causing a wide range of pelvic health issues such as dryness, itching, increased need to pee and urgency to pee.

Pelvic health concerns can be a barrier to exercise, as the fear of incontinence and increasing the risk of an 'accident' is understandable. Your pelvic floor muscles respond to training in the same way that your other skeletal muscles do. The good news is that it's never too late to improve your pelvic floor, and pelvic floor muscle training is a valuable way to address this.

In addition to incorporating pelvic floor muscle training to strengthen the pelvic floor, we need to be mindful of how other exercises can either help or hinder the pelvic floor. How you coordinate your breath, with either relaxing or bracing the core and pelvic floor, is an important aspect of strength training. We will look at this in more detail in Chapter 6.

Exercise to support immune function

Physical activity plays an important role in influencing immune function in several ways. The frequency, duration and intensity of your workout matters, though. Studies suggest that moderate to vigorous activity for 60 minutes or less is optimal for immune function, whereas prolonged high-intensity exercise with insufficient rest can suppress the immune system.

Dr Jenna Macciochi explains further:

'Regular physical activity enhances thymic function, preserving the thymus's ability to produce vital T cells that are essential for robust immune responses. Exercise mitigates unwanted inflammation by reducing pro-inflammatory cytokines and promoting anti-inflammatory ones, balancing the body's inflammatory response.'

The effects of physical activity on immune function have been highlighted in several studies, including one that involved a group of cyclists aged 55–79. The researchers discovered that the study subjects, who had maintained a high level of physical activity throughout their lives, had immune profiles akin to younger individuals. The cyclists had higher levels of T cells, crucial for immune response, and a more active thymus.

The study concluded that physical inactivity with age can be an important driver of immunosenescence, reduced thymic output and lower levels of regulatory T cells.[13]

Our aim as an active ager is to engage in sufficient exercise to support the immune system, recognise the impact inactivity can have on immune function, and balance this with sufficient recovery time in order to avoid illness.

CHAPTER 5

THE BIG LIFE CHANGES

As I entered my fifties the spread of ages in my children meant they had very different needs. My eldest son, who was 25 at the time, was busy setting up a business; my eldest daughter, then at the age of 20, needed financial and emotional support whilst at university; my middle son was studying for his A levels; my youngest daughter was studying for her GCSEs and my youngest son was in his final year of primary education and preparing for his SATs. Life was stressful, as I was being pulled in every direction. I was juggling teenage angst, exam stress, worrying about my daughter away at university, concerned about my own menopause symptoms, and then amid all this my husband was made redundant.

Big life events often collide in midlife and they have the potential to derail our physical health and psychological wellbeing. Changes in personal circumstances, like divorce or the end of a relationship, redundancy and moving home, can all have a significant impact on your mental health and your body.

Women are often the middle in the sandwich between ageing parents, who may have their own health issues and require increasing levels of support, and older but still financially dependent children.[1]

Dr Charlotte Ord conducted her doctoral research on midlife and shares her thoughts on this.

'It's noticeable how the media often portrays this period of life in a negative light; midlife crisis, self-doubt, physical decline, asexuality (especially for women), empty nest syndrome, etc., and yet it can also be a period of reflection and subsequent liberation as women are freed from their

parenting duties and have more opportunity to focus on what they really want, whether that be personal development, relationships, hobbies or career goals.'

Although I'm in my sixties now, I am still the middle in the sandwich. This is what happens when you have five children and an age gap of 14 years between your oldest and youngest! My youngest is finishing his final year of university, and when he leaves and hopefully finds employment it will be the first time in 30 years that my husband and I won't have children who are financially dependent on us. At the same time my parents are in their eighties, live independently in their own home, but in recent years they have both started to experience some health problems. Fortunately, they live a short distance from me; I can walk to their home in under 5 minutes. Which is reassuring for them and me, as increasingly my help is being called upon. As my only sibling Jonathon died many years ago, I carry the burden of worrying about my parents' future needs alone.

I recognise I am experiencing anticipatory grief. If you have ageing parents, or are caring for someone with a terminal illness, you may have similar feelings. Watching my parents grow older makes me acutely aware of their mortality.

Anticipatory grief is the grief we feel before someone actually dies, and it's accompanied by myriad emotions, like fear, sadness and uncertainty. Not everyone will experience this, and there's no right or wrong approach. Some may find optimism, holding on to hope and focusing on the present moment is a helpful coping strategy when faced with the prospect of losing a loved one. Others might imagine confronting the situation will help them better prepare themselves to let go when the time comes.[2]

If you're caring for an ageing parent, or you are in an unpaid caring role for a family member, you are not alone. In the UK, women are far more likely to become carers than men; with 58 per cent of women in an unpaid caring role. And in women aged between 55 and 59 years old, 20 per cent provide unpaid care. With the average age of women giving birth in England and Wales increasing, and life expectancy also increasing, more women are and will become sandwich carers – caring for older, sick or disabled relatives as well as dependent children. This can place a huge toll on a woman's physical and mental health, with 27 per cent of sandwich carers showing symptoms of poor mental health.[3, 4, 5]

Caring responsibilities aside, a huge number of women will also face the emotional and financial cost of divorce in their forties and fifties. The average age for divorce is 43.9 for women in the UK, 44 per cent of couples who married in 1987 are now divorced, and an estimated 50 per cent of marriages will have failed by the time couples reach their fifties. Women tend to see their household income drop significantly following a divorce, with research suggesting this drop can be as much as a third. Women who have been cohabiting with a partner may find themselves even worse off after a split, as only jointly owned assets are included in a financial split unless a cohabitation agreement is in place.[6, 7]

Children are staying in the family home longer and later in life, with over six in ten 20 to 34-year-olds living with their parents.

Data from Census 2021 indicates a continuing upward trend of more adult children living at home with one or both parents.

There are several factors that most likely explain this trend, not least of all the cost of suitable housing, unemployment and adult children providing unpaid care.[8, 9]

My own grown-up children have all needed to stay in our family home after completing their studies at university, another two to four years each. This has been down to the unaffordability of rental properties, despite all gaining employment in their chosen careers straight after graduation.[10, 11]

When grown-up children start their own families, many midlife women find themselves further stretched, physically and financially, by providing unpaid childcare. Around 80 per cent of grandmothers take care of a grandchild under the age of 16. Whilst many women do this willingly, and love spending time with their grandchildren, the knock-on effect can mean a depleted state pension through reduced contributions, less or non-existent hours in paid employment, a drop in income and minimal free time to look after their own health and needs.[12, 13]

Divorce, bereavement, redundancy, grown-up children still living at home, becoming a carer for an older relative or providing childcare to grandchildren; big life events and circumstances like these are common in midlife. They can have a significant impact on our physical and psychological health as well as our financial wellbeing.

Adjusting to new life circumstances can be tricky. I have become adept at defining and maintaining my boundaries. This includes ring-fencing my time for exercise and giving priority to things that really matter to me. I don't take on work-related projects that encroach on family time, or reply to emails on weekends. As I've got older, I have found it easier to say no without feeling the need to explain my decision.

You may get some push back when setting your boundaries, especially if family, friends or work colleagues have got used to you being at everyone's beck and call. This can be uncomfortable at first, as Dr Charlotte Ord acknowledges.

'Prioritising self-care might mean having to lean into difficult feelings like guilt, or tough thoughts such as being selfish, but this is key to protecting your own health and ensuring that destructive feelings such as resentment don't manifest. None of us can pour from an empty cup, and you can only give the best of yourself to others if you are well looked after yourself.

'Other people often dislike change, especially if it goes against what they would like. Their feelings are theirs to work through, not your responsibility. Accept that it might take time or be a bit bumpy, and keep reiterating your boundaries.'

Making health and fitness a priority despite these pressures, financial concerns and being time-poor, is a challenge for active agers. But I strongly believe we can, and we must. We have to break the cycle of women in midlife who experience poor and deteriorating health, who then rely on younger relatives or adult children for care in later life, because, as we have seen, most of these carers are women. Women providing care in their fifties and sixties, with little time to focus on their own needs today, are at risk of becoming the women who need care tomorrow.

Which is why in the exercise guides in this book I have included time-saving workouts, with minimal equipment. So, whether you are time-poor, need a workout you can do in an older relatives' home, or don't have the spare cash to buy lots of fitness equipment, there are workouts you can follow here.

CHAPTER 6

YOUR PELVIC HEALTH

Perhaps you are wondering why I have dedicated an entire chapter to pelvic health, and how it is relevant to active ageing. But the structures and muscles in your pelvic area are every bit as important as the skeletal muscles, joints and bones in the rest of your body, and they are also subject to the physiological effects of ageing. Pelvic health issues can be a significant barrier to exercise; I am only too aware of this through the conversations I have with my clients, as well as my followers online. This chapter will help you understand exactly what structures and muscles are involved in your pelvic region, the effects of ageing on them, how to support your pelvic health, and recognising the signs of dysfunction and what to do about it.

I'm going to hazard a guess here and bet that most of us were not taught about pelvic floor anatomy, or what pelvic floor health refers to, at the same time we learned about menstruation and puberty. This is not a reflection on our mothers or caregivers, it's likely they didn't receive any education on this either.

The first time I heard about the pelvic floor was when I was pregnant with my son, at the age of 26. I can remember my antenatal teacher referring to exhaling and allowing the pelvic floor muscles to relax during labour. After my son was born, I was given a sheet of paper, in with my hospital discharge notes, with instructions for a few postnatal exercises to strengthen stretched abdominal muscles. Among the instructions was a note that simply said: 'Remember to do your pelvic floor exercises.' I'd had an episiotomy, which had extended into a large tear during my son's birth. I had no idea where my pelvic floor was for at least a week! This was the extent of pelvic floor health education, and support, given to new mothers in 1989.

I would like to think that this situation has changed in the intervening years, and that nowadays women receive greater information, education and support on pelvic health matters. This important topic is not only relevant for women during and after pregnancy, but all women regardless of whether they've ever given birth. I certainly believe things are improving, and one way to tackle this is to start having these conversations with girls at a younger age.

Guidelines issued by NICE in 2021 are an attempt to address this, aiming to raise awareness in women over the age of 12 to reduce the risk of pelvic floor dysfunction.[1]

The Royal College of Obstetricians and Gynaecologists (RCOG) is also calling for action to reduce the number of women living with poor pelvic health, through improving education and providing timely support.[2]

Clare Bourne, a specialist pelvic health physiotherapist and author of *Strong Foundations: Why Pelvic Health Matters*, endorses the need to extend pelvic health education to all.

'Pregnancy and childbirth are just two risk factors for pelvic floor dysfunction symptoms. The truth is that they can impact anyone of any age, any gender, and there are lots of different risk factors, including chronic constipation, chronic cough or respiratory conditions and genetic factors.'

After my third bout of Covid during the pandemic I can testify to the potential impact of a chronic cough on the pelvic floor. Fortunately for me this was a short-term issue, but it has helped me appreciate one of the risk factors for pelvic floor dysfunction. Several studies have looked at the link between COVID-19 and pelvic health, and it has been hypothesised that respiratory symptoms of Covid, including coughing, could contribute to new or worsening pelvic floor function, including incontinence and pelvic organ prolapse.[3]

This was certainly borne out in recent research that found 38 per cent of women who were already experiencing some symptoms of pelvic floor dysfunction noticed a worsening of their symptoms during the pandemic.[4]

Before we go any further, this pelvic floor health checklist will help you identify potential red flags. It's something I run through with new clients (alongside the Physical Activity Readiness Questionnaire (PAR-Q), which we will look at in the next chapter) to make sure exercise prescription is safe and effective and to avoid any exercises that may make a pelvic floor health issue worse. For example, it's important to avoid exercise that involves jumping movements or very heavy weights if urinary incontinence is an issue, as both may increase the risk of leaking.

1.	Are you having trouble with your bowel, wind or urinary urges?	Yes	No
2.	Do you lose urinary control when laughing, sneezing, coughing or jumping or moving quickly?	Yes	No
3.	Are your bowel movements or urination painful?	Yes	No
4.	Do you experience a sensation of pressure in your vagina or rectum, or have you noticed any protrusions from your orifices? Has anyone ever said you may have a prolapse?	Yes	No
5.	Are you incontinent overnight?	Yes	No
6.	Do you currently, or have you ever, needed to wear incontinence pads?	Yes	No
7.	Do you suffer from constipation or regularly strain on the toilet?	Yes	No

If you answered yes to any of these pelvic health checklist questions, please don't continue to suffer in silence. A doctor will be able to offer advice or refer you for further tests, if necessary. Answering yes to any, or some, of these questions suggests you may have a pelvic floor health issue, or you could develop one. For example, if you regularly experience constipation this increases your risk of developing haemorrhoids and can in some cases lead to a prolapse. Alternatively, you could seek a referral to a pelvic health physiotherapist.

Clare Bourne explains further.

'I help patients with a wide range of symptoms, including bladder symptoms (urinary incontinence, urgency or frequency of passing urine), bowel symptoms (faecal incontinence, constipation and wind constipation), sexual symptoms (pain with intercourse and loss of pleasure with incontinence) and persistent pelvic pain, as well as pregnancy related pelvic girdle pain.'

It's understandable to feel worried, apprehensive or embarrassed if you have pelvic health issues. The pelvic floor health checklist has enabled me to identify numerous clients who may need further support with their pelvic health and encourage them to see their GP or pelvic health physiotherapist.

Anna, who was struggling with stress incontinence, shares her experience of working with a pelvic health physiotherapist.

'My initial consultation involved a detailed conversation where I talked about my symptoms and the scenarios where I was most likely to experience stress incontinence. Rose, my pelvic health physiotherapist, immediately put me at ease and explained how my pelvic floor muscles work.

'There was no pressure to have a physical examination, but Rose explained how this can aid assessment of the abdominal muscles, pelvic floor muscles and vaginal wall. This helped me understand the benefits of the assessment, and how this would enable Rose to offer me more detailed guidance on addressing the stress incontinence I was experiencing. So I went ahead with the physical assessment and felt reassured with Rose's findings and recommendations.'

Your pelvic floor health matters at whatever age you are. Any issue with your pelvic floor can have a direct impact on your physical and mental wellbeing, as well as your ability to engage in and enjoy exercise. It has particular importance to us as active agers; it's common for problems to arise as we get older. Some of these issues are due to hormonal changes as well as sarcopenia, which affects all our muscles as we age, including our pelvic floor muscles.

Pelvic floor muscles can be affected by many things during a woman's lifetime, including body weight, chronic constipation, a chronic cough or bronchitis, lack of exercise, pregnancy, labour and family history. Sometimes it's the accumulation of these factors, alongside the hormonal changes of menopause, that contribute to pelvic health issues in midlife.

The toiletries aisle of every supermarket is stocked with an extensive range of incontinence pads, which gives an indication of the demand for these products. Whilst pelvic floor issues like prolapse and incontinence are incredibly common, 'common' should never be confused with normal. Gendered ageism persists in the assumption that all old women smell of urine. Previous generations of women believed stress incontinence, and prolapses, were an inevitable part of getting older. We now have the education and strategies to prevent and manage pelvic floor health throughout our lifespan.

Clare Bourne explains further.

'It is never too late to build and work on muscles, so doing pelvic floor rehabilitation can really help. Though we might think of pelvic floor muscle training as purely improving the strength of muscles, exercises also help with improved blood flow to the tissues of the vulva and vagina, as well as improving overall pelvic floor function and flexibility, and tissue elasticity in postmenopausal women.'

Pelvic structures

Let's be clear what structures are involved in your pelvic health before we go any further.

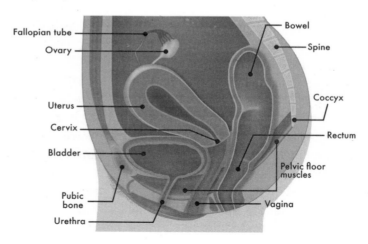

Your pelvic area includes the fallopian tubes, ovaries, uterus, cervix, bladder, bowel, urethra, rectum, pelvic floor, vulva and vagina.

From an exercise and physical activity perspective we are primarily focused on:

- The bladder
- The bowel
- The pelvic floor.

The bladder

A normal healthy bladder expands and stretches to accommodate the storage of urine. As it becomes fuller, the brain receives signals that the bladder is approaching capacity, so that you know to take yourself to the toilet. Once you have urinated, the bladder contracts down and starts the process all over again. This continues throughout the day.

The bowel

The bowel consists of two parts – the small bowel and the large bowel – and is part of the digestive system. The small bowel sits between the stomach and the large bowel. Its role is to break down food and allow the absorption of vitamins, minerals and nutrients. Once food has passed through the small bowel it continues to the large bowel. The large bowel removes water and nutrients before expelling the waste products as poo.

The pelvic floor

The pelvic floor muscles are often referred to as a hammock, and support the bladder, uterus and bowel. These muscles attach to the bony structure of the pelvis at the front, back and sides, and are made up of a superficial layer and a deeper layer. From an aerial view imagine these pelvic floor muscles like two doughnuts, or a figure of 8, with rings circling the urethral and anal sphincters.

Your pelvic floor has five main functions:

1. Support: Supports the bladder, bowel and uterus against gravity and downward pressure.
2. Stability: Stabilises the spine and pelvis, along with other muscles that make up the inner core.

3. Sphincteric function: The sphincters open to allow urine and faeces to be excreted from the body, and help prevent leakage of urine, faeces and wind.
4. Sexual function: Plays a role in orgasm and sexual pleasure, but can also be a source of painful intercourse.
5. Circulation: Acts as a 'sump pump' to circulate blood and lymph from the pelvic region and back towards the heart.

The other inner core muscles

Your pelvic floor works alongside other muscles, referred to as the inner core muscles. These inner core muscles are the diaphragm, transversus abdominis and multifidus. These work together to stabilise the spine and pelvis during movement and at rest.

The diaphragm

This muscle assists with breathing, moving air into and out of the lungs. It sits underneath the ribcage and above the pelvic organs.

Transversus abdominis (TVA)

This acts as a corset for the trunk, wrapping around the body from the spine and meeting in the middle of the abdomen.

Multifidus

This isn't just one muscle but multiple muscles, as the name implies. These long, narrow muscles are located either side of the spine and assist stabilisation.

Imagine these muscles of your inner core as a can or cylinder. Your diaphragm sits at the top, the multifidus at the back, the transversus abdominis circling around from the spine to the front, and the pelvic floor is at the bottom. During inhalation the diaphragm contracts and flattens downwards, the transversus abdominis expand and the pelvic floor lengthens and relaxes. On exhalation the diaphragm

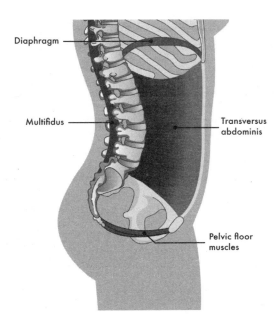

Diaphragm

Multifidus

Transversus abdominis

Pelvic floor muscles

relaxes and lengthens, moving upwards, the transversus abdominis contracts and the pelvic floor lifts upwards and contracts.

Pelvic health issues

Understanding how these muscles work together, and what can go wrong, is relevant to your pelvic floor health, your daily life and is pertinent to exercise.

Intra-abdominal pressure

The inner core muscles create and respond to movement by creating pressure. Pressure is lower for some activities or when sedentary, and higher for other activities. If intra-abdominal pressure is a new concept to you, the feeling when this pressure increases will be very familiar because this is what happens when you empty your bowels, especially if you strain. To locate your transversus abdominis and increase intra-abdominal pressure, push your fingertips gently into your abdomen, a few centimetres either side of your tummy button. Now cough once and feel how the muscles under your fingertips (the TVA) quickly tighten, as the pressure in your abdomen increases. If you've ever experienced leakage of urine when you cough, this is why. When intra-abdominal pressure increases abruptly, like a sudden cough, downward pressure on the pelvic organs and pelvic floor increases. If the pelvic floor muscles aren't strong enough the urethral sphincters fail to contract sufficiently, and an involuntary loss of urine follows. This is known as stress incontinence and if you've experienced this you may have noticed it also occurs at other times, like when you laugh, lift something heavy or if you run or jump. We will revisit intra-abdominal pressure, the pelvic floor and exercise considerations in the fitness section. Understanding how these work together will ensure you avoid creating downward pressure on your pelvic floor, decreasing the risk of stress incontinence during exercise.

Incontinence

Incontinence is a common problem, and the true scale of it is hard to assess as it's still a bit of a taboo topic. Many people are embarrassed to discuss incontinence or seek medical help. Some studies estimate that 14 million people in the UK experience urinary incontinence, and half a million people have faecal incontinence. Increasing age is associated with higher levels of faecal incontinence, with 15 per cent of adults over 85 who live at home affected by it. This figure is thought to be higher in nursing homes, with some studies suggesting 50 per cent of residents in care homes may experience both urinary and faecal incontinence.[5, 6]

A recent survey reveals the worrying number of women in the UK who have pelvic health issues and don't know how to address this, with one in five experiencing urinary incontinence, one in four affected by urge incontinence, over half who don't do pelvic floor exercises, and a quarter who don't know how to do them.

If you're affected by pelvic health issues this next section will help you recognise the symptoms, inform you how to perform pelvic floor exercises and indicate when you might need to seek help.[7]

Many people think incontinence refers to the involuntary leaking of urine, but it also refers to incontinence of the bowel.

There are several types of urinary incontinence, including stress incontinence (for example, when you sneeze and wee), urge incontinence (for example, when you experience an urgent need to wee as soon as you put your key in the door but struggle to make it in time), and an overactive bladder (for example, urgency to pass urine, which is hard to control during the day and night).

Bowel incontinence includes urge incontinence and passive incontinence. Urge incontinence is characterised by a sudden urge to empty the bowels, but leakage occurs before you're able to get to the toilet. Passive incontinence is characterised by a lack, urge or awareness of when leakage occurs, as well as soiling in underwear.

Any type of incontinence is distressing and can impact your physical health as well as your mental wellbeing. It can affect your sexual pleasure and intimacy with significant others, as well as everyday activities and exercise. It can make you reluctant to stray far from home, and anxious when travelling. You may feel self-conscious at work or in social gatherings and stressed about drawing attention to yourself with frequent bathroom visits.

Pelvic organ prolapse

Pelvic organ prolapse refers to the movement downwards of one or more of the organs in the pelvis – namely the vagina, uterus, bladder, bowel and rectum. It's thought that one in four women in their forties, and one in three in their sixties are affected by prolapse.[8]

There are several reasons why a prolapse may develop, and risk factors include pregnancy, childbirth, genetics, excess body weight, constipation or a persistent cough.

Unlike incontinence, where the symptoms are more obvious and you are likely to know if you experience this, you may not always recognise the symptoms suggestive of a prolapse. These include:

- Heaviness around the lower abdomen and vagina.
- The sensation that something is inside the vagina.
- Feeling like you are sitting on a small ball.

- Unable to empty the bladder completely.
- Difficulty emptying the bowels fully.

Pelvic health issues and solutions

Now you understand more about the structures in the pelvis and what can go wrong, let's look at solutions and how you can help yourself. These include:

- Diaphragmatic breathing.
- Pelvic floor exercises.
- Coordinating breathing and pelvic floor contraction/relaxing with exercise.
- Seeking specialist help from a pelvic health physiotherapist.
- Surgery may be considered if non-surgical options have not worked or a prolapse is more severe.

Diaphragmatic breathing

We all know how to breathe – we do it every day without thinking about it. Yet we don't always breathe deeply, we sometimes hold our breath and we may not focus on what's happening to our pelvic floor as we are breathing.

Diaphragmatic breathing helps you connect to how the diaphragm moves during inhalation and exhalation, as well as how to feel and visualise how the pelvic floor responds.

Practise diaphragmatic breathing by:

1. Lying face up on your bed or an exercise mat.
2. Place the palm of one hand flat, splaying your fingers against the rib cage, and place the other hand flat against your abdomen.
3. Take a deep breath in and focus on allowing your rib cage and abdomen to expand underneath your hands.
4. At the same time, imagine how your pelvic floor is lengthening and relaxing as your vagina lets go of any tension.
5. Try this for several breaths.

Once you are happy with diaphragmatic breathing from a lying position, try practising from a side-lying position, as well as standing. This can be helpful to practise at any time to reconnect with your breath and as an aid to relaxation.

Pelvic floor exercises

Like many other muscle groups in your body, the pelvic floor muscles include fast-twitch and slow-twitch muscle fibres. Fast-twitch muscle fibres respond quickly to contract the pelvic floor, like during orgasm, or to stop the leakage of urine when you sneeze. These muscles tire easily. Your slow-twitch muscles provide constant tone to support your pelvic organs, even when you are asleep, and tire slowly. When performing pelvic floor exercises, we need to train both the fast-twitch and slow-twitch muscle fibres.

Before we try to target these different muscle fibres, let's run through this exercise while lying down. This is the easiest position in which to practise pelvic floor exercises initially, as you are not trying to contract the pelvic floor against gravity.

Lie down and relax your arms at your sides. Once you feel settled, take a deep inhale and, on the exhale, start to squeeze and lift your back passage (anus), as though you are trying to stop wind escaping. Then continue and extend the squeeze, working from the back passage towards your front passage (vagina). Imagine the muscles around your front and back passage drawing upwards like a lift going up several floors. As you exhale gently, release this contraction, lowering the lift back downwards. During this exercise focus on keeping your buttocks and tummy muscles relaxed. Practise this several times.

Now try to repeat the same exercise again from a seated position, then from a standing position. You may find this exercise challenging at first, so stick with practising from a lying-down position if you feel this is the most effective way for you to perform a pelvic floor exercise.

If you are comfortable kneeling down on the floor and sitting back on your buttocks, this is another way to practise a pelvic floor exercise. Before you sit back on your buttocks, wedge a cushion under your groin and between your thighs, so that you are sitting astride it. Perform the pelvic floor contraction by exhaling, squeezing and lifting your back passage away from the cushion. Then extend this contraction through to the front of your pelvis and the vagina. You should feel like you have created some space underneath the cushion now. As you exhale and gently release the contraction you should once again feel the cushion beneath you as the gap narrows. The ability to be able to relax and release the pelvic floor is as important as the contraction and release, so give both phases equal attention.

Once you are confident you know how to perform a pelvic floor contraction, it's time to vary the type of contraction you do to target the fast-twitch muscle fibres and the slow-twitch muscle fibres.

Slow long contractions (targeting slow-twitch muscle fibres)

The aim is to hold the contraction for several seconds whilst breathing normally. Start with relaxing and inhaling, then as you exhale initiate the pelvic floor contraction, squeezing and lifting from the anus through to the vagina. Maintain this contraction as you continue to breathe normally in and out. At first you may only be able to hold this contraction for a few seconds, but with practice aim to build up to 10 seconds at a time.

Fast–quick contractions (targeting fast-twitch muscle fibres)

The aim is to fully contract and squeeze, followed by releasing quickly. Think of these as fast but strong pulses. Try to do several in a row, 5–7 to begin with, building up to 10.

It's important to target both slow- and fast-twitch muscles to support your pelvic floor health, so ensure you include both types of contractions – slow, long contractions and fast, short contractions.

Pelvic floor contractions are very effective and help many women, but only if you remember to do them! I have performed lots of pelvic floor contractions whilst writing this chapter, I suspect you have been doing them too as you've been reading. It's easy to remember to do something when we are being prompted to do so – like seeing an advert for something and adding it a shopping list. Here's a prompt I used to recommend when I taught antenatal classes many years ago, and still recommend clients to do the same thing. Ideally, you want to practise pelvic floor exercises several times a day, every day, for life. So, link pelvic floor exercises to something else you do regularly during the day, like every time you put the kettle on or brush your hair. Alternatively, you could try putting sticky notes in several places throughout your home to act as a visual reminder. Back in the 1990s, when I was teaching ante-natal classes, we didn't have mobile phones or apps, but nowadays you can download an app to your phone that will prompt you to remember to do your pelvic floor exercises.

A good number to aim for is 10 slow contractions followed by 10 fast contractions, 10 times a day.

Whilst pelvic floor exercises and physical activity can both assist pelvic health, Clare Bourne also advises:

- *Treat any constipation: Straining can weaken our pelvic floor tissues and be linked with bladder and prolapse symptoms.*
- *Speak to your doctor about vaginal oestrogen: A small amount of oestrogen to the vulval and vaginal tissues can really help improve bladder, vaginal and vulval symptoms, such as bladder urgency and frequency, recurrent UTIs, vaginal dryness and pain with intercourse.*
- *See a pelvic health physiotherapist: we can help treat symptoms, make a long-term plan for your pelvic health, and explain how specific devices may help you.*

Despite our very best efforts to address a pelvic health issue, through all the measures we have covered in this chapter, problems can persist. Should you find yourself in this situation please don't assume you are destined to spend the rest of your life wearing incontinence pads. Whilst there is nothing wrong with pads for comfort, dignity and reassurance, there are alternative lines of treatment to consider.

Conservative management may not work for everyone, but if you haven't had tailored advice from a pelvic health physiotherapist then this is worth exploring before considering surgical options.

Clare Bourne says, '*We often advise trying physiotherapy for at least 3–6 months and exhausting all conservative approaches prior to considering surgical options.*'

In the exercise chapters we will look at how we link pelvic floor contractions and breathing to specific movements and exercises. In daily life we need our pelvic floor to work effectively when we are moving around and whilst engaging in structured exercise, not just when we are standing or sitting still and thinking about it. I hope this chapter has helped you understand the importance of your pelvic floor health, its relevance to exercise and ageing, how you can help yourself or who to seek help from, and why your pelvic floor exercises need to be a lifelong daily habit from this day forwards.

CHAPTER 7

HOW TO EAT WELL

What you eat and drink plays an important role in how you feel and function at any age. Nutrition affects every aspect of our health and wellbeing. A nutrient-dense diet provides an extensive range of vitamins and minerals, which are essential for hundreds of functions in the body. Unhealthy diets in the UK are estimated to lead to over 75,000 premature deaths each year, whereas improving dietary quality has the potential to extend both health span and lifespan.

As an active ager we need to be especially mindful of how food fuels our workouts, aids performance, promotes recovery post training and supports the retention of lean muscle and healthy bones. We need to be aware of and respond to changes in nutritional needs as we grow older. For example, preserving muscle mass, which naturally starts to decline with age, requires a sufficient intake of dietary protein, as well as engaging in regular strength training.

Part 1: Food basics

In this next section I'm going to cover some key information about the food you eat. This will either serve as a useful recap, if you are familiar with the constituents of food, or help further your understanding of food and nutrition and how it influences health.

The food you consume is made up of three macronutrients: carbohydrates, proteins and fats. Macronutrients are required in large quantities for energy, and for the efficient functioning of systems in the body and its structure. Micronutrients refers to vitamins and minerals. These are required in smaller quantities, relative to macronutrients. Although your body requires fewer of these micronutrients, vitamins and minerals are critical to health and a deficiency can have serious consequences.

We don't eat macronutrients and micronutrients, though, we eat food! When you consume food, it is rarely made up of a single nutrient, but instead often contains a mix of nutrients. Before nutrients in food can be absorbed, they need to be broken down. In simple terms, carbohydrates are broken down into sugars, proteins are broken down into amino acids, and fats are broken down into fatty acids.

Your nutritional needs are individual to you. There is no 'one-size-fits-all' approach to nutrition. Instead, the optimal intake of each macronutrient and micronutrient for you is influenced by multiple factors, including your age, activity levels, gender, genetics and your metabolism. There are some general principles that apply to everyone, though. Before we look at the bigger picture, let's look at these macro- and micro-nutrients more closely.

Carbohydrates

Carbohydrates are used in the body as a source of energy. After consuming a meal the carbohydrate content is converted to glucose, which is then used as energy or stored as glycogen to be used at a later date.

There are two main types of carbohydrates: simple carbohydrates and complex carbohydrates. In general, complex, unrefined carbs are of greater nutritional value than simple carbs.

Starchy, fibre-rich complex carbs include potatoes, wholegrain bread, cereal products, rice and grains and pasta. Fruits, vegetables, legumes, nuts and seeds are also carbohydrate food sources.

Simple carbohydrates contain sugars and refined grains, which are less nutritious. Examples of simple carbs include biscuits, cakes, crisps and white bread.

Protein

Protein is an essential macronutrient, made up of building blocks called amino acids. It's used in the body to build and repair muscles, skin, hair and nails. Proteins also enable numerous metabolic functions to take place in the body.

Protein is obtained from plants and animal sources, including red meat, eggs, fish, chicken, turkey, milk, nuts and seeds, as well as beans and pulses. The body requires nine essential amino acids in order to work efficiently, and the number of amino acids available from different protein sources varies. Foods that contain all nine amino acids, in sufficient amounts, are known as complete proteins. Plant sources of protein don't contain all nine essential amino acids and are known as incomplete proteins. As a result, vegans and vegetarians benefit from combining proteins and eating a wide variety of proteins, to ensure they obtain all the essential amino acids.

Fat

Fats are an important macronutrient used in the body for storing energy, the protection and cushioning of organs, and the absorption and transportation of fat-soluble vitamins A, D, E and K. Consuming sufficient fats is necessary for many functions in the body, such as brain health, which requires the essential fatty acid omega-3.

There are two types of fats – saturated and unsaturated. Unsaturated fats are either monounsaturated fats (MUFAs) or polyunsaturated fats (PUFAs). MUFAs are usually liquid at room temperature, such as olive oil and nut oils. Nuts and seeds are also a good source of MUFAs. PUFAs can be found in oily fish, walnuts, flaxseed and vegetable oils.

Saturated fats are normally solid at room temperature, and mainly come from animal sources. Sources of saturated fats include milk, cheese, red meats, processed meats, cakes and biscuits. It's recommended to keep saturated fats to a minimum, as diets high in saturated fats are linked to heart disease.

Trans fats are unsaturated fatty acids. They are present in small quantities in natural sources. However, they are more commonly used as an additive to prolong shelf life, and are made from hydrogenated cooking oil using heat and pressure. This process enables the oil to be solid at room temperature. This industrially produced trans fat is found in margarines, fried foods and baked products such as biscuits and pies.

The UK government has urged food companies to cut down on the use of trans fats. This is due to the wide range of health issues associated with consuming trans fats, which are known to increase cholesterol and the risk of developing heart disease, strokes, liver dysfunction, type 2 diabetes and Alzheimer's disease.

Due to these serious health consequences the World Health Organization recommends adults should limit the consumption of trans fat in the diet to less than 1 per cent of energy intake.[1]

Fibre

Fibre is the indigestible part of carbohydrate. It's found in plants, the skins and seeds of fruits and vegetables, nuts and wholegrains. Fibre helps the passage of waste materials through the intestine and helps keep the digestive system healthy. Foods that are high in fibre also help us feel fuller and can prevent constipation.

There are numerous positive health outcomes from consuming fibre, but many of us don't eat enough of it. The current recommendation is that adults should consume 30g of fibre a day, but the average person in the UK only consumes 20g.[2]

There are two types of fibre – soluble and insoluble. A well-balanced diet includes a mixture of both. Soluble fibre dissolves in water and is found in foods like beans, peas, oats, apples and citrus fruits. Insoluble fibre doesn't break down, is found in beans, wheat and bran, green beans, potatoes, cauliflower and nuts. As insoluble fibre doesn't break down, and is only partially broken down during digestion, it helps aid the movement of waste products through the digestive tract.

Starch and fibre are sometimes confused. Both are carbohydrates, but starch can be broken down by enzymes in the digestive system.

Vitamins

Vitamins are nutrients contained within food. They are referred to as a micronutrient, along with minerals, because we only require them in small quantities. Vitamins are organic substances, made by plants or animals, and are essential to a healthy functioning body. If you consume a wide variety of foods in your diet, you are more likely to obtain all the vitamins you need. However, vitamin deficiencies can occur in some restrictive diets, during times of ill health when appetite may be affected, and in diets that are devoid of fresh foods.

In general, if you consume a wide variety of foods it is not necessary or advisable to take a multivitamin supplement 'just in case', or to top up your vitamin intake. This is because some vitamins can be dangerous if consumed in excess or can cause unpleasant side effects like an upset tummy and digestive issues.

Vegans and vegetarians may need to be especially vigilant to avoid vitamin deficiencies, though. This can be overcome by consuming specific plant sources with key vitamins. Obtaining enough vitamin B12 in a vegan diet can be particularly challenging, as it is only found in animal products and in some fortified plant foods.

Sometimes vitamin supplementation may be beneficial or necessary. For example, vegans who find it difficult to get enough vitamin B12 in their diet may need to take a B12 supplement. In the UK, adults are generally advised to take a vitamin D supplement during the winter months. Vitamin D is known as the sunshine vitamin because this is made when skin is exposed to the sun, however, in the UK the sun isn't strong enough and we don't get enough of it to make sufficient vitamin D from September/October through to March/April.[3]

A vitamin D test is generally advised before you start to supplement, to ascertain the correct supplement dosage. Your doctor can normally do this for you, or you can carry out a home test.[4] This is something I send off for and complete on an annual basis. The test is very simple to do; the package contains a blood spot collection card and everything you need to supply four pin-prick samples of blood, which you then send back to the laboratory. You'll receive your results a short time afterwards, and an explanation about what to do next, depending on your results.

Types of vitamins

There are two types of vitamins, known as water-soluble vitamins and fat-soluble vitamins. Water-soluble vitamins dissolve in water and are mainly B vitamins and vitamin C. They cannot be stored in the body so they need replenishing frequently. Whereas fat-soluble vitamins A, D, E and K are not required daily as these can be stored in the body.

Water-soluble vitamins

B vitamins play an important role in keeping the nervous system healthy and help release energy from the food you consume.

Vitamin B – roles and sources

Vitamin	Role	Source
B1	Helps turn food into energy and keeps the nervous system healthy	Peas, bananas, nuts, wholegrains, fruit, liver
B2	Helps break down proteins, fats and carbohydrates	Eggs, milk, rice, fortified breakfast cereals, mushrooms
B3	Helps turn food into energy, keeps the nervous system healthy, fights fatigue and helps to keep skin healthy	Meat, fish, eggs, milk
B5	Helps turn food into energy, and assists the production of cholesterol and steroid hormones	Chicken, beef, eggs, dairy, porridge, potatoes
B6	Plays a role in mood and brain and immune function, creating haemoglobin and neurotransmitters	Meat, fish, lentils, eggs, bananas, peanuts, oats
B7	Helps the body make fatty acids. Supports the nervous system, liver, eyes, skin and hair	Only required in trace quantities but present in a wide range of foods
B9	Helps make red blood cells, reduces the risk of neural tube defects in unborn babies	Green leafy vegetables, chickpeas, some fortified breakfast cereals, broccoli
B12	Helps make red blood cells, keeps the nervous system healthy, use folate and release energy from food	Only found in animal products and some fortified breakfast cereals

Vitamin C helps to protect cells in the body, keeping them healthy. It's also important to help maintain healthy skin, blood vessels, cartilage and bones. Vitamin C is necessary for wound healing and helps the absorption of iron.

Vitamin C – role and sources

Vitamin	Role	Source
C	Growth and repair of cells, healing wounds, maintenance of healthy skin, blood vessels, cartilage and bones	Citrus fruits, peppers, broccoli, bananas, strawberries

Fat-soluble vitamins

Fat-soluble vitamins are important for several functions in the body, including cell repair, bone health, wound healing and healthy skin.

Fat-soluble vitamins – roles and sources

Vitamin	Role	Source
A	Assists with cell renewal and repair	Cheese, eggs, oily fish, liver, peppers and carrots
E	Helps maintain healthy skin	Almonds, avocados, plant oils, nuts, seeds
D	Helps the body absorb calcium and supports bones and muscles	Present in small quantities within food, including egg yolks, red meat, oily fish. Made from skin exposure to sunlight
K	Important for wound healing and essential for blood clotting	Green leafy vegetables, broccoli, spinach, vegetable oils

Minerals

Minerals are inorganic elements that originate from soil and water. Plants absorb and animals consume these inorganic elements, which we then obtain in our diets when we consume vegetables, fruits and meat products.

We require some minerals in greater quantities and others in smaller quantities. Minerals are classified accordingly into major or macro minerals, and trace or micro minerals. The major minerals include calcium, phosphorus, chloride, magnesium, potassium and sodium. Trace minerals include iodine, iron, selenium, zinc, copper, fluoride and manganese.

Minerals – roles and sources

Mineral	Role	Source
Calcium	Important for healthy bones and teeth	Dairy products, green leafy vegetables, bread made with fortified flour
Phosphorus	Builds and maintains healthy bones and teeth	Dairy products, oats, bread, fish, meat
Magnesium	Helps food into energy, assists in nervous system function and muscle contractions	Nuts, cereals, bread, green vegetables
Potassium	Helps control the balance of fluids in the body and is important for blood pressure	Potatoes, bananas, beans and pulses, nuts and seeds, beef, fish, chicken, turkey
Sodium chloride (salt)	Helps balance body fluid levels	Salt is found naturally in many foods at low levels. Salt is also an additive in numerous processed foods*
Iodine	Assists in the making of thyroid hormones and normal thyroid function	Fish, dairy products, eggs, some plant foods
Iron	Necessary for red blood cell production, carrying oxygen around the body, helps immune and brain function	Liver, red meat, beans, nuts, dried fruits
Selenium	Helps the immune system and helps prevent damage to cells and tissues	Fish, Brazil nuts, eggs, meat
Zinc	Assists the immune system and hormone production, helps process food	Eggs, red meat, cheese, shellfish, chickpeas
Copper	Helps produce red and white blood cells, also assists in triggering the release of iron to form haemoglobin	Nuts and shellfish
Fluoride	Helps prevent tooth decay	Found in trace amounts in a variety of foods. Commonly added to dental products like toothpaste
Manganese	Helps make and activate some of the enzymes in the body, which assist in a range of chemical reactions, like breaking down food	Bread, nuts, green vegetables, wholegrain cereals

*Most people are consuming too much salt, with the average in the UK being 8g (3.2g of sodium) against a daily recommendation of no more than 6g (2.4g of sodium).

Hydration

Hydration is an essential element of nutrition. Water is key to numerous vital functions in the body. This includes your blood, which transports essential nutrients, oxygen and glucose around the body, your kidneys to filter out waste products, the efficient functioning of your digestive system and to keep your eyes, joints and skin healthy.

Water is also important to your brain, as dehydration can lead to confusion, an inability to concentrate and can also affect mood. Each day the body loses water during these various functions, as well as through perspiration and excretion.

The food you eat contributes to 20 per cent of your fluid intake. The remainder needs to come from water or other drinks. Although sugary drinks, fruit juices and caffeinated drinks contribute to total fluid intake, it's best to limit your intake of them. These often contain other ingredients that are not helpful to health when consumed in excess, like sugar and caffeine.

How much water do you need?

Perhaps you've heard a recommendation to drink eight glasses of water a day, but this isn't based on scientific research, it in fact dates to 1945 when the US Food and Nutrition Board of the National Research Council recommended that adults should consume 64 ounces of fluid a day. Fluid can be obtained from food and drinks, not just water. However, the original recommendation was misinterpreted, so that the advice became that everyone everywhere should consume eight glasses of water a day. Although this is easy to remember, it doesn't consider your gender, body size, physical activity, exercise, climate, temperature and lifestyle.

How to check your hydration status

If you don't consume enough fluids you can quickly become dehydrated. Dehydration has negative effects on how your body functions, and signs of dehydration include tiredness, dizziness, headaches, confusion and dry mouth, lips and eyes. Checking your urine colour is a simple way to assess your hydration status. When you are well hydrated urine is pale and clear, whereas urine is darker in colour when you are dehydrated and has a stronger odour.

Hydration and ageing

Ensuring you are well hydrated may also help you live longer and reduce your risk of developing a chronic disease, according to a study from the National Institutes of Health.

The study followed 11,000 adults, who were between the ages of 45 and 66 at the start of the research, over a 30-year period. To determine hydration status the researchers looked at sodium levels in the blood, as higher levels indicate a poor hydration status. The researchers found that study participants who had higher levels of sodium faced an increased risk of ageing faster, as they were more likely to be assessed as biologically older, develop chronic diseases and die at a younger age.

The study findings are interesting, but it's important to understand the difference between causation and correlation. Causation means that one thing causes another, while correlation identifies a relationship between one thing and another. In this research the study showed a strong correlation between dehydration and faster ageing, the development of chronic disease and earlier death.[5, 6]

Increasing age is also associated with a blunted thirst mechanism, which in turn increases the risk of dehydration. One study has shown up to 40 per cent of older adults may be chronically dehydrated. This may be due to this less sensitive thirst mechanism or prescription medications that cause dehydration. In some cases deliberate reduction of fluid intake in adults, who are concerned about incontinence, may result in dehydration too.[7, 8]

The key takeaway points as an active ager are:

- Drinking eight glasses of water a day is a general recommendation; a better figure to aim for is somewhere between 1.5 and 2 litres per day.

- On days when you are very active, in warmer weather or you are sweating a lot, you may need to increase your fluid intake.
- Monitoring your urine and making sure it is pale and clear in colour, not dark, is a simple way to check you are not dehydrated.
- You may not be able to rely on feeling thirsty to indicate dehydration as you get older, so make sure you consume sufficient fluids so that your urine remains pale and clear.

Part 2: What is a healthy diet?

In this next section we will discuss how to build a healthy diet, and in doing so we will consider energy requirements and activity levels. Body weight can be an emotive topic, but we will touch on weight-management strategies and menopausal changes in body fat distribution if this is something that concerns you.

There is an abundance of information around about healthy eating and what a balanced diet looks like. Despite this, it seems like every week a new type of diet gains popularity. Nutrition is often in the news as well, either because there are fresh claims surrounding the benefits of a particular food, or (more often) reports about potential negative effects of a foodstuff. There's a lot of dogma surrounding the benefits of some diets, and many people are left thoroughly confused about what to eat and what not to eat.

It's important to keep in mind that there is no perfect diet that suits everyone. Many factors influence what will determine a good diet for you. Your ideal diet is guided by your needs, food likes and dislikes, activity levels, lifestyle, beliefs, location, personal finances, current health status and whether you have any medical conditions.

Despite personal preferences and factors that may influence your dietary choices, there are key principles that are beneficial to everyone. A healthy diet should include a range of different sources of carbohydrates, proteins and fats. Variety is considered important for gut health.

Rather than focus on one meal, it might be easier to think about the range of food you eat in a day, and then over a course of a week. There are two things to consider: firstly, the proportion of carbohydrates, proteins and fats. Secondly, eating a range of foods from each food group.

The Eatwell Guide from Public Health England recommends the following each day:[9]

- Five portions of a variety of different fruits and vegetables (more vegetables than fruits).
- Three to four portions of starchy carbohydrates (wholegrain where possible).
- Two to three portions of protein (beans, pulses, fish, eggs, meat).
- Two to three portions of dairy or dairy alternatives (low-fat and lower-sugar options).
- Small amount of fats like unsaturated oils.

Researchers have quantified the impact on life expectancy when changing from unhealthy dietary patterns to the Eatwell Guide dietary recommendations. They have shown that sustained dietary adherence to the Eatwell Guide is associated with an increase in life expectancy of 8.9 and 8.6 years, for 40-year-old men and women respectively.[10]

How to measure a portion

Food packaging often suggests portion sizes. Another simple method is to use your hand to estimate portion size as follows.

1 portion =
- Fruits and vegetables – 1 fistful
- Starchy carbohydrates – 1 cupped handful
- Protein – 1 palm-sized amount
- Dairy – 1 thumb-sized amount
- Fat – 1 thumb-sized amount

Energy balance

Energy balance refers to the relationship between energy in and energy out. Energy is obtained, in the form of calories, from food and drink you consume, which your body uses each day to perform essential functions like breathing and digestion, as well as movement, which includes everything from brushing your teeth to structured exercise.

When energy in equals energy out, body weight remains the same. If energy in exceeds energy out, weight is gained; but if energy in is lower than energy out, weight loss occurs.

Body-weight terminology

Body weight, body size and shape can be highly emotive topics. If you have a good relationship with food and are happy with the skin you are in, you are blessed. Unfortunately, many women spend a lifetime locked in a battle with their body, often trying to conform to a societal ideal of size or shape in pursuit of the 'perfect' form.

In recent years the body positivity movement has helped promote body diversity and greater acceptance of different shapes. The term 'larger body' is sometimes substituted for those who may be defined clinically as 'overweight' or 'obese'. This can avoid the stigma often associated with these terms.

Whether body weight is something that you feel you need to address or not, I have good news for you – exercise is beneficial even when body weight remains exactly the same. In those classified as 'overweight' or 'obese' (in a larger body) research has shown physical activity improves various health markers, even in the absence of weight loss.[11]

Weight management

If your body weight is of concern to you, you may find the concept of 'weight management' more helpful than 'weight loss' – as the latter has a strong association with quick fixes and restriction, and can perpetuate an unhealthy relationship with food. Weight management, on the other hand, doesn't tie you to a specific numerical goal on which success or failure hangs.

Think of weight management as a range with an upper and lower end where you feel comfortable and believe this is realistic and achievable for you. You may have a desire to stay within this range but appreciate there are times when you'll be at the upper end and other times when you'll be at the lower end. To do this you might implement long-term strategies, lifestyle behaviours and dietary approaches in order to avoid big fluctuations in body weight and yo-yo weight gain and loss.

Factors that influence body weight in midlife

The hormonal changes around menopause affect where we store excess fat in the body. Prior to menopause, excess weight is more often stored around the hips and thighs, but after menopause we tend to store more fat around the waistline and abdomen. This is known as visceral fat, which is more dangerous than subcutaneous fat because it lies inside the abdominal cavity and wraps around internal organs. Some studies have shown that, on average, visceral fat increases from 5–8 per cent pre-menopause to 15–20 per cent post-menopause. Any increase in visceral fat can have a potentially adverse effect on health, which includes an increased risk of cardiovascular disease.[12]

There are several reasons why visceral fat and body weight increases during menopause, besides the hormonal changes. These include reduced activity levels, the ageing process, poor sleep and other lifestyle factors.

Short sleep duration can be especially problematic for successful weight management, as it is significantly associated with obesity. This is mostly down to two hormones that signal hunger (ghrelin) and fullness (leptin). Various research studies have shown that sleep directly influences the level of these hormones. In addition, sleep disruption impacts stress response and an increase in cortisol levels – which is also linked to weight gain.[13, 14]

It's important to note that the energy balance equation is still relevant to women in menopause and beyond; excess body fat can only be gained in an energy surplus. If you feel you need, or want, to lose weight, it's necessary to create an energy deficit – in other words, you need to increase energy expenditure and decrease energy intake. The directive 'eat less, move more' oversimplifies the energy deficit equation, because what remains in our diet when we 'eat less' is important, and how we move matters.

Fat loss is an extremely complex and nuanced topic. Environmental factors, social factors, genetics, medications, disabilities and race all influence body weight. Some people have a higher baseline appetite and are more susceptible to weight gain as a result. Recent research has shown a key region of the brain involved in controlling appetite, the hypothalamus, differs in people in larger bodies (who are classified as overweight or obese) when compared to those whose weight is classified as healthy. Whilst this research only proves a relationship, not the cause, it highlights the need for greater understanding about the complexities of why some people struggle with weight gain.[15]

To be clear, when we are talking about weight loss we mean reducing body fat levels without losing lean muscle. If we drop our energy intake from all food groups equally, we risk losing more than fat mass.

I had this exact problem when I competed in my first bodybuilding competition. I recall a friend in the gym commenting about my butt shrinking. I'd successfully stripped body fat to quite low levels, so my muscles were more clearly defined for the competition, but in the process my glutes (butt) had lost a bit of muscularity.

Even if you have no intention of taking part in a bodybuilding competition, it's important to focus on maintaining the optimum intake of one macronutrient – protein – to reduce fat mass without losing precious muscle, which is already under threat and declining as we grow older.

Movement in the form of strength training will help ensure the maintenance of your lean muscle mass, alongside consuming sufficient protein. 'Eat less' normally requires a reduction in carbohydrates, especially sugars and refined carbohydrates, rather than protein.

The UK guideline for women is to consume 0.75g of protein per kilogram of body weight. For a woman who weighs 60kg this would be 45g of protein, the equivalent of two portions of meat, fish, nuts or tofu a day. However, these guidelines are considered a minimum, and they don't take into consideration your level of activity. Some research points to protein intakes of 1.4–2g per kilogram per day being beneficial for physically active individuals, especially if you are engaged in strength training.[16]

The timing of your meals is also relevant to weight management. The popular phrase, 'eat breakfast like a king, lunch like a prince and dine like a pauper', coined by a medieval philosopher Maimonides centuries ago, would appear to have merit. A growing body of evidence suggests that meal timing can have a direct impact on body weight.[17]

Your sleep–wake cycle over a 24-hour period is influenced by circadian rhythm. This 24-hour clock influences many other systems in your body, including the nervous system and digestive system, as well as the production and secretion of hormones. Numerous studies have shown a link between eating later in the day, increased weight gain, abnormal appetite and higher levels of stress.

Your body systems are optimised to process and digest the food you eat in daylight hours. So it isn't just what you eat, but when you eat that can influence body weight. Shifting your pattern of eating to consume your largest meal at the beginning of the day may be worth considering if you are struggling with weight management and if weight loss is your goal.

Weight-management strategies

There are several different ways to approach weight management and reducing body fat. These broadly fall into two methods: either a tracking or a non-tracking approach. Tracking is a numerical approach to monitoring your energy intake of food and drink and/or energy expenditure of physical activity. This involves counting, calculating and recording:

- Calorie intake
- Macronutrients
- Protein
- Exercise
- Steps per day.

A non-tracking approach doesn't involve counting and instead tends to rely on the following principles:

- Intermittent fasting
- Time-restricted eating
- Plate size and portion control
- Eliminating specific foods
- Eliminating alcohol.

It's beyond the scope of this book to go into each of these in detail. However, let's expand on calories, as an awareness of energy expenditure is relevant to active ageing even if we don't need or want to track calories.

Calorie counting

The only time I have counted calories was when I was a competitive bodybuilder, and I found it incredibly tedious and not always accurate! However, many people find this to be a helpful weight-management strategy. In addition, it can be a useful educational tool, bringing greater awareness to food choices and how this impacts energy intake. Other people may find it stressful, and something that triggers an obsessive and unhealthy relationship with food.

Before we go any further, let's just clarify what calories are. A calorie is a unit of energy used to measure the energy content of food and drink. When you expend energy during exercise this can also be measured in calories. You can find out the calorie content of food by looking at food labels, checking with online nutrition resources, or using an app. Protein and carbohydrates contain 4 calories per gram, whereas fats contain 9 calories per gram.

If you think tracking calories might be helpful for you, there are many apps to make this simpler. Fitness trackers and wearable devices provide you with a wealth of information and data, many of which enable you to log food and activity, and will provide you with information on step count, heart rate, sleep and body temperature. Just keep in mind any information you obtain from these devices is intended as a guide. They can be inaccurate and are not foolproof.

I enjoy wearing my fitness tracker, and I have found it always detects an elevation in my usual resting heart rate (RHR) when I am ill, which is accurate as we know RHR tends to increase in response to infection, illness and stress. I don't use it to log calories 'burned' or food consumed, though. Instead, I find the fitness data it gives me in terms of distances travelled, heart rate training zones and tracking workouts useful.

Calculate your calorie requirements

If you want to track the calories you eat in order to support weight management, it's important to know your daily calorie requirement alongside your daily energy expenditure; these are known as BMR – basal metabolic rate – and TDEE – total daily energy expenditure.

BMR – basal metabolic rate

Your basal metabolic rate is the number of calories your body uses every day just to function. There are several different formulas we can use to estimate BMR, but below is the Mifflin–St Jeor equation, which the American Council on Exercise (ACE) recommends. You can use this to work out your own BMR or use one of the online calculators.

> **Women BMR =**
> (10 × weight in kg) + (6.25 × height in cm) – (5 × age in years) – 161
> **Men BMR =**
> (10 × weight in kg) + (6.25 × height in cm) – (5 × age in years) + 5

Here's an example for a 50-year-old woman called Nicole, who weighs 60kg and is 168cm tall.

> **BMR =**
> (10 × 60kg = 600) + (6.25 × 168cm = 1050) – (5 × 50 = 250) – 161
> 600 + 1050 – 250 – 161 = 1239

In this example Nicole requires 1239 calories each day for her body to perform the most basic life-sustaining functions.

This example goes some way to explain why the 1,200-calories-a-day diet is not sustainable for most women.

Since as far back as 1918, a 1200-calorie-a-day diet for women has been popularised. The origin of this diet is thought to stem from the book *Diet and Health with Key to Calories* by Lulu Hunt Peters, MD, which was published in the same year. If you've ever attempted a 1200-calorie-a-day diet, and either struggled to maintain it or found you lost some weight but then your weight plateaued, your BMR requirement is key to understanding why. Most women will require at least 1200 calories a day for basic life-sustaining functions, and while a very low 1200-calorie-a-day diet can lead to fat loss, it needs to be followed consistently for it to work. What tends to happen is people can sustain this diet for a few days, but then, driven by hunger cues, will overconsume calories on other days, increasing daily average calories. Your BMR drives behaviour; your body wants you to survive and not simply to have enough calories for life-saving functions!

TDEE – total daily energy expenditure

To calculate your total daily energy expenditure, you need to factor in your physical activity level (PAL).

Use this table as a guide to assess what best describes your current level of activity.

Activity level	PAL
Sedentary lifestyle with little activity	1.2
Light activity (1–2 days per week)	1.375
Moderately active (3–5 days per week)	1.55
Very active (6–7 days per week)	1.725
Extremely active (6–7 days per week)	1.9

Let's use Nicole as an example again. Nicole drives to her office-based job five days a week, she attends a Pilates class once a week after work and likes to meet up with her friend on alternate Saturdays for a 3-mile walk, so long as it isn't raining. On this basis Nicole's activity level can be described as light, she has a mostly sedentary lifestyle due to her office-based job and she's involved in light activity for 1–2 days each week.

TDEE = BMR × PAL
Nicole's TDEE = 1239 × 1.375 = 1704 calories

Based on Nicole's BMR and activity level she needs 1704 calories a day to maintain her current body weight.

If Nicole consistently consumes more than 1704 calories, she will be in an energy surplus and will gain weight. Likewise, if she consistently consumes less than 1704 calories, she will be in an energy deficit and lose weight.

To reduce body fat

Calculating your BMR and TDEE is only necessary if your chosen weight-loss method relies on tracking calories.

A good rule of thumb is to start with reducing your daily calorie intake by 500 calories. This will amount to 3500 calories over seven days, which roughly equals 0.5kg of fat loss each week. This means reducing your TDEE by 500 calories. Removing 500 calories from your diet every day can be challenging; an alternative approach is to combine increasing your levels of physical activity with reducing calories consumed. A 50:50 approach works well for many people – reducing energy intake by 250 calories and increasing energy expenditure by 250 calories. The cardiovascular and circuit workouts in this book will all contribute around 250 calories to your daily energy expenditure.

Keep in mind that when you lose body fat and your total body weight reduces, you need to recalculate your BMR and TDEE, as both will decrease. This effectively means you need to keep reducing energy intake to match any weight loss. This is partly why it can feel easier to lose weight at the start of a weight-loss journey but gets progressively harder to sustain.

In conclusion, if you want to reduce body fat levels, focus on achieving your dietary protein requirements every day first, as well as ensuring your diet follows the principles outlined in this chapter.

Part 3: Eating for ageing

In this final section we will look at specific dietary approaches that are known to be beneficial for health conditions often associated with increasing age. Even in the absence of illness how we eat as we are ageing can either support healthier ageing or increase the likelihood of developing a chronic disease.

Eating a well-balanced, healthy diet is important at any age and something we really need to pay attention to as we grow older. The risk of developing chronic diseases increases with age. We can take steps to reduce these risks through everything we've covered so far in this book, but our approach to nutrition matters as well. For example, consistently eating in an energy surplus increases the risk of becoming obese, which is linked to an increased risk of heart disease, type 2 diabetes and cancer.

Let's briefly consider some key issues with an ageing body, and how diet can play a role, before looking at some specific dietary approaches in more detail.

Heart health

The risk of developing cardiovascular disease increases with age, especially post-menopause. Aside from exercise, cardiovascular health is supported by reducing saturated fats, eating a high-fibre diet, limiting salt to less than 6g a day (approximately 1 teaspoon) and eating plenty of fresh fruit and vegetables.

Brain health

Our brains, much like the rest of our body, rely on nutrients to function efficiently. When asked what her number one tip for brain health is, Dr Lisa Mosconi, world-renowned neuroscientist and author of *Brain Food*, replies, '*Do not eat processed foods.*'[18]

Even if we weren't already aware of a link between brain health and processed foods, we can't fail to be aware of the association between increasing age, cognitive decline and ultimately dementia.

There is a growing body of evidence that suggests a link between brain processes and specific nutrients in foods. Cognitive function in older adults is positively influenced by foods containing omega-3 fatty acids, flavonoids, vitamins B, D and E and choline.

There is also increasing interest in how dietary patterns, rather than specific foods, may influence brain health. A world-leading research project funded by Age UK, called the Disconnected Mind, has been looking at the effects of diet on the brain. The study is measuring the brain volume of Scottish people over time. The project so far has gathered dietary information from the cohort at the age of 70 and scanned their brains at 73, 76 and 79 to look at the differences in brain volume over time. It has discovered that those who do not follow a Mediterranean diet (see page 112) are more likely to exhibit a higher loss of total brain volume.[19]

Some degree of brain shrinkage over time is common in older adults, even in those without cognitive impairment. One area of ongoing research is to look at whether specific dietary patterns can slow down brain atrophy, and whether this in turn will be protective against cognitive decline.

Bone health

Bone mineral density decreases with age and is more pronounced post-menopause. To offset this loss, and to promote healthier bones, it's vital to consume sufficient quantities of calcium. Most adults require 700mg of calcium each day, which can be obtained by eating a well-balanced diet that includes calcium-rich foods such as dairy products, green leafy vegetables, almonds, pulses and fortified foods. For those who already have osteoporosis, and older adults, the general advice is to increase calcium intake to 1000mg per day.

Vitamin D is also important to bone health, as it helps your body absorb and use calcium. As we learned earlier in this chapter, vitamin D is obtained by exposure to sunlight, in small quantities from food and through supplementation.

Muscle health

Maintaining healthy muscles and joints can become challenging as we grow older. Muscular atrophy refers to the shrinking and wasting away of muscles. This can be because of age, malnutrition, genetics and some medical conditions. Any loss of muscle has the potential to impact daily function, so taking steps to preserve your muscle mass is a priority as you get older. Diet plays a role, alongside physical activity, to support the retention of lean muscle. Adequate protein consumption helps maintain, repair and build muscles, but increasing protein intake alone is not sufficient.

In a recent meta-analysis of older adults (mean age ≥ 50), the effect of increasing protein intake combined with regular resistance training resulted in increases in lean body mass and hand grip strength.[20]

In addition, as we get older our bodies require considerably more protein. Studies have repeatedly shown that older adults need to consume 25–30g of protein three times a day to stimulate muscle protein synthesis – the process by which the body maintains and builds muscle. Based on this, the recommendation is to aim for a palm-size portion of protein at each mealtime.[21]

Joint health

Although osteoarthritis isn't an inevitable consequence of growing older, it is very common in older adults. Osteoarthritis is a degenerative joint condition that causes swelling and pain, and can affect range of movement in a joint. Some 73 per cent of people who have osteoarthritis are over 55, and 60 per cent of these are women. Typical onset occurs during the late forties and early fifties, during perimenopause and menopause.

If you have osteoarthritis, the most significant dietary intervention is maintaining a healthy body weight to avoid and reduce excess loading on joints. A recent umbrella review set out to look at the evidence for any specific dietary approaches. It found that most evidence supports a Mediterranean diet, which is considered 'anti-inflammatory', and associated with improvements of common symptoms such as pain, stiffness and inflammation, the biomarkers of cartilage degeneration.

Dietary approaches for health and longevity

The following diets are not diets in the way we have come to think of them. Diets have become synonymous with weight loss, food restriction and calorie counting for a defined period of time. Instead, these diets are about a way of eating for life, to either benefit general health as we grow older or address a specific health problem associated with increasing age. These dietary approaches bring a shift in focus to foods that are beneficial to add into our diets, rather than those to take away. The word diet in this sense is more closely linked to how it was first used in English language in the thirteenth century, to mean *habitually taken food and drink.*[22]

The Mediterranean diet for general health

The Mediterranean diet has its origins in the countries that surround the Mediterranean Sea as well as parts of the world where olive trees grow and is the eating pattern and traditional foods, including olives and olive oil, of people who live in southern Spain, Italy and Greece.

The Mediterranean diet focuses on food quality and consists of an abundance of fresh and plant-based foods, as well as wholegrains, oily fish and lean poultry. Healthy unsaturated fats, predominantly from olive oil, are an integral part of the Mediterranean diet.

Although no foods are banned, those wishing to gain the health benefits of a Mediterranean-style diet reduce their consumption of red meats, sweets, full-fat dairy products and processed foods.

The health benefits to those who follow a Mediterranean diet have been highlighted in numerous studies. These include reducing the risk of developing several chronic conditions such as cardiovascular disease, type 2 diabetes, high blood pressure and high cholesterol. It's also an eating pattern associated with increases in both health span and lifespan. These health benefits are thought to be due to high levels of monounsaturated fatty acids and polyphenols derived from olive oil, polyunsaturated fatty acids from fish, and many anti-oxidants present in fruits, vegetables and legumes.[23]

A recent study has also shown the protective effective against long-term cognitive decline in older adults who adhere to a Mediterranean diet.[24]

So even if you don't have joint issues such as osteoarthritis or joint pain, which is often a symptom of menopause, following a Mediterranean-style diet can still be beneficial to overall health.[25]

Whereas some dietary approaches can be confusing and very rigid, the Mediterranean diet is generally considered one of the easiest to follow. This is because it doesn't have a set of rules, and instead follows principles that are simple to implement, regardless of your lifestyle.[26]

Here are some suggestions as to how you can move towards this dietary pattern.

- Fill half your plate with a range of different vegetables for a minimum of two of your daily meals.
- Aim for three servings of fish a week that are high in omega-3 fatty acids.
- Other proteins to include are lean poultry (in moderation), eggs and plant-based sources of protein, including legumes and nuts.
- Choose minimally processed wholegrain foods.
- Make extra virgin olive oil your main source of dietary fat.
- Snack on fruit or vegetables.
- Flavour food with fresh herbs and spices.
- Reduce consumption of red meats, sweets, full-fat dairy products and processed foods.

The Blue Zones diet

Why some people live longer, healthier lives is a matter of considerable scientific interest. In 2004 Dan Buettner, in association with National Geographic and the National Institute on Aging, and joined by a team of researchers, set out to identify areas in the world where people live longer and explore the reasons why this is so. These areas became known as Blue Zones and include Ikaria in Greece; Loma

Linda in California; Nicoya in Costa Rica; Okinawa in Japan; and Sardinia in Italy. In August 2023, a sixth Blue Zone, Singapore, was added to the list.[27, 28]

In comparison to the rest of the world, a disproportionate number of people living in Blue Zone areas reach the age of 100, and there is less chronic disease in the general population. In short, residents of Blue Zones live longer, healthier lives than anywhere else in the world.

Dan Buettner, National Geographic and teams of scientists then set out to identify what lifestyle characteristics might explain health and longevity in Blue Zones. In all, they identified nine specific traits. As you might expect, diet plays an important role and this is one of the nine specific traits, referred to as Eat Wisely. Although the diets of each Blue Zone area differ, Dan Buettner and the team picked up common approaches to eating, which include the 80 per cent rule and plant slant.

The theory behind the 80 per cent rule is that people who live in Blue Zones stop eating when they are 80 per cent full, tend to eat their smallest meal of the day in the late afternoon or evening, then don't eat anything else before bed. Plant slant refers to the people who live in Blue Zones who consume a vast amount of locally grown vegetables, as well as a variety of different beans, so that plants make up 95 per cent of their diet. People in four of the five original Blue Zones do eat meat, but they do so sparingly.

Unsurprisingly, two of the Blue Zones – Ikaria and Sardinia – follow a Mediterranean diet.

You may not have heard of the following two diets, the DASH diet and the MIND diet, despite them being well-researched with overwhelming evidence of their benefits. Unfortunately, GPs are often unable to refer patients for dietary support on how to implement these diets due to a lack of funding.

The DASH diet to lower blood pressure

The Dietary Approaches to Stop Hypertension (DASH) diet was developed in the 1990s to see if specific dietary interventions could be used to treat hypertension (high blood pressure). It was developed by a team of researchers, funded by the National Institute of Health, who were tasked with studying whether specific dietary interventions could be helpful in treating hypertension.[29]

What is blood pressure?

Cardiovascular fitness was one of the physical components of fitness we looked at earlier in this book. Cardiovascular fitness is defined as the ability of the heart and blood vessels to supply nutrients and oxygen to tissues and muscles throughout the body. This process is seriously compromised by high blood pressure, which damages artery and blood vessel walls.

Heart disease is a result of the build-up of fatty deposits, known as plaque, in the coronary arteries. The arteries become stiff and harden, which reduces blood flow to the heart muscle and can weaken and damage it.

Blood pressure is measured as two numbers:

1. Systolic: The first number is a measure of the amount of pressure your blood exerts on artery walls when the heart beats.
2. Diastolic: The second number is a measure of the amount of pressure your blood exerts on artery walls while the heart rests between beats.

Blood pressure and age

With an ageing population, rising rates of obesity, sedentary lifestyles and poor dietary choices, more people are at risk of developing hypertension in their lifetime than ever before. It poses a serious risk to health, can lead to strokes, heart disease and renal disease, and is a major cause of premature death worldwide.[30]

In the UK, 30 per cent of adults have hypertension, and the prevalence increases by age. In over 65s this figure rises to 60 per cent of adults, which means your chance of developing high blood pressure in your lifetime rises to roughly one in three by your mid-sixties. In the US it's a similar story, with 30 per cent of the adult population having hypertension, and 2000 people dying each day because of heart disease.[31]

Although in theory I should be at a lower risk of developing hypertension, due to my lifestyle and diet, I don't take my blood pressure for granted. As many as 4.2 million adults in the UK are estimated to have undiagnosed high blood pressure, including, it's thought, nearly 30 per cent of women between the ages of 55 and 64.[32]

I monitor my blood pressure through taking regular readings at home with a reliable blood pressure monitor. If you want to do the same, it's recommended you use a device that is UK approved, and validated for accuracy, by the British and Irish Hypertension Society (BIHS).

The large prevalence of undiagnosed high blood pressure is also part of the reason why personal trainers, like me, will take a blood pressure reading of a new client during the initial health screening process. Personal trainers are not qualified to give medical advice or reach a diagnosis of high blood pressure – only a doctor can do this – but the screening process enables us to pick up a potential problem with blood pressure (and other red flags) and refer a client to a doctor, where necessary, before commencing exercise.[33]

Whilst medications are available to treat hypertension, following the DASH diet has been seen to have a positive effect on blood pressure. It has long been recognised that addressing lifestyle factors like the foods we eat, taking regular exercise and reducing stress are crucial in managing blood pressure.

The DASH diet study found specific dietary interventions resulted in decreasing systolic blood pressure by 6 to 11mm Hg. This was observed in both those with pre-existing hypertension (high blood pressure) and those with blood pressure in the normal range.

If your blood pressure is creeping upwards, your doctor is monitoring this during regular check-ups and you've been advised that medication could be necessary in the future, the DASH diet may be something to consider and discuss with your doctor. Some doctors may not be aware of this dietary treatment, as many are not trained in nutrition. It is worth being prepared for this eventuality and asking for a referral to a dietitian who can support you in following the DASH diet.

Priya Tew, dietitian and author of *The Dash Diet*, advises:

'The research does suggest that when the DASH diet is combined with a low salt intake it can have a beneficial effect on blood pressure, and medication may be avoided. It can be a first line intervention to try out for a limited period (four weeks is a good time) and then review with a doctor.'

Foods prominent in the DASH diet include vegetables and fruit, lean meat, dairy products and minimally processed food. It follows heart-healthy strategies to limit saturated fats and trans fats, and instead focuses on foods that contain nutrients known to lower blood pressure – like potassium, calcium and magnesium, as well as protein and fibre. It also reduces sodium in the diet to 1500 mg/day. The DASH diet has been the subject of many clinical trials and has been shown to not only lower blood pressure but also to lower LDL cholesterol, reduce the risk of strokes, cardiac events and the development of type 2 diabetes. It's also a helpful dietary approach for losing weight and maintaining a healthy weight.[34]

It has also been seen to have a positive effect in decreasing bone turnover and improving bone mineral density – an important consideration for women post-menopause.[35]

DASH foods fall into these groups:

- Wholegrains
- Vegetables
- Fruits
- Fat-free or low-fat dairy
- Lean meat and fish
- Nuts, seeds and legumes
- Fats and oils.

DASH food serving suggestions are also critical to the DASH diet. This is an approximate outline of the proportion of each food group, but the serving sizes and amounts of each will vary according to your daily energy requirement.

DASH food	Servings
Wholegrains	5 per day
Vegetables	5 per day
Fruits	5 per day
Fat-free or low-fat dairy	2 per day
Lean meat and fish	2 per day
Nuts, seeds and legumes	2–3 per week
Fats and oils	Small amount

With the estimated number of people who have undiagnosed high blood pressure, alongside those who are already receiving treatment and an ageing population who are at greater risk of developing high blood pressure, Priya offers these final thoughts on how to implement the DASH diet.

'I'd recommend making what feels like simpler switches, then if that works make some more switches. Focus on cooking from scratch at least one day a week, swap a snack a day for a serving of nuts, and stop adding salt to meals.'

The MIND diet to support brain health

The Mediterranean–DASH Intervention for Neurodegenerative Delay (MIND) diet was designed by nutritional epidemiologist Dr Martha Clare Morris, in 2015, to target brain health in older adults with an aim to reduce the risk of dementia and cognitive decline. It includes elements of the Mediterranean and DASH diets.

The MIND diet contains foods that are thought to protect the brain by reducing inflammation and oxidative stress. Martha Clare Morris and her colleagues identified ten foods that are associated with brain function and lowering the risk of Alzheimer's. Each of the ten foods are rich in compounds that have been shown to protect and nourish brain health.

Just like every other organ in your body, your brain needs energy to work, which is obtained from the food and drink you consume. The brain uses 2 per cent of the calories you obtain each day, at rest, to carry out its daily functions. The neurons that make your brain work need nourishment and depend on the quality of the food you eat for the many complex jobs that your brain does.

The brain determines which nutrients it will allow in, and which it will block entry to via something known as the blood–brain barrier, a semi-permeable membrane. Just like every other system in the body, this blood–brain barrier ages and needs help to function well as we grow older.

Dr Morris's MIND diet foods include:

- Green leafy vegetables
- Wholegrains
- Berries
- Nuts
- Beans
- Vegetables
- Fish
- Poultry
- Olive oil
- One glass of wine (5oz) a day.

Dr Morris and her colleagues then created a diet score system for each of these food items, which was used in The Memory and Ageing Project study, which assessed the dietary intake of these MIND foods with residents in retirement communities.

The results of this study showed that the participants with the highest MIND food scores had a younger cognitive age than those with lower MIND food scores. This amounted to 7.5 years difference in cognitive age between the highest and lowest scores. No one on the study achieved the optimal MIND food score, which suggests improvements to cognitive age can still be made by including some of the ten MIND foods.

MIND food serving suggestions

MIND food	Servings
Green leafy vegetables	6 or more per week
Wholegrains	3 or more per week
Berries	2 or more per week
Nuts	5 or more per week
Beans	More than 3 per week
Vegetables	1 or more per day
Fish	1 or more per week
Poultry	2 or more per week
Olive oil	Primary oil used
Wine	1 glass a day

The MIND diet has been the subject of many other studies since Dr Morris's original research.[36, 37, 38, 39] The results of these do point to a positive link between the MIND diet and cognition in older adults. However, science is still some way off from giving us definitive answers and eliminating the risk of developing dementia and Alzheimer's based on diet alone. As it stands, most dementias are thought to be caused by several factors, and food is just one piece of the puzzle.

Based on current information and the other known health benefits associated with foods included in the MIND diet, it may still be prudent to consider this dietary pattern or move towards it whilst understanding further research is required.

These dietary approaches are all slightly different but there are some consistent themes – prioritising whole grains, eating an abundance of fresh vegetable and fruits, and choosing lean protein sources – including beans, nuts and healthy fats. Whereas processed foods, sweets, baked goods and saturated fats are either non-existent or kept to a minimum.

If you are left wondering where to begin (for you or your family), here's something to contemplate.

In the UK, only 29 per cent of adults eat five or more portions of fruit and vegetables a day, and 7 per cent eat no fruit or vegetables at all. It can feel overwhelming to move towards a healthier way of eating if our diet deviates a long way from optimal, but changing this one thing – eating more vegetables and fruits – could be a significant step in the right direction for 71 per cent of adults in the UK, providing a healthy mix of nutrients and a good place to start.[40]

Eating for exercise, before and after

Your daily energy intake, and achieving your macronutrient and micronutrient requirements, matters more than the precise timing of when you eat. Keep in mind we have already covered how eating larger meals earlier in the day and smaller meals later in the day is linked to better overall health.

How you eat around exercise can be driven by your personal preferences, your schedule and what works for you. For the most part, I prefer to exercise first thing in the morning, at sunrise, which can be very early in the summer months. Consequently, I don't eat before I train, because I am not hungry, and because I don't want to wait an hour or more for my food to go down before exercising. My first meal of the day is anywhere between an hour or two after waking, and sometimes as many as 3–4 hours. I'm not suggesting you need to follow this approach; this is just something that suits me and fits with my schedule.

There is some scientific evidence for avoiding eating immediately on waking, though. This is due to the hormone melatonin. The level of melatonin in your blood is highest at night, decreases during daylight hours, and plays a role in your sleep–wake cycle. There is growing interest in the connection between melatonin and blood glucose control, and studies show that eating too close to bedtime or too soon after waking can be disruptive. Many studies have suggested a cut-off time of eating somewhere between 2 and 3 hours before going to bed, then waiting an hour after waking before eating anything. This will ensure melatonin levels are optimal and won't be detrimental to glucose control.[41]

Whilst I don't tend to eat before I exercise, I do prioritise refuelling after my workouts with carbohydrates and protein. Carbs are converted to glycogen, and your body uses this to fuel workouts. If your glycogen stores are low, this can affect your ability to exercise, and your performance. If you're not training first thing in the morning, try to eat a meal two hours before training. Aim for this to be mostly carbohydrate-based, with some protein and a small amount of healthy fats. If you intend to exercise straight after you finish work you'll most likely benefit from a snack beforehand. Eating a banana or a home-made cereal bar an hour before you leave work will give you some much-needed energy to power through your session.

General guidelines on what to eat before a workout

Here are some general guidelines on eating and drinking before your workout:

- Ensure you are well hydrated before you start.
- If you intend to exercise within an hour of eating, choose foods that are easy to digest and not too heavy.
- A small snack that contains carbohydrates would be ideal, such as a banana or low-fat yogurt.
- Foods high in fibre or fat take longer to digest, so these are best avoided.
- When you have 2–3 hours between eating and exercise, a food combination of some slow-release carbohydrates and lean protein would be beneficial, such as wholegrain rice with a skinless chicken breast and mixed vegetables.

General guidelines on what to eat after a workout

Refuelling post workout can help recovery, by replenishing glycogen stores, providing protein to support muscle protein synthesis and support rehydration – especially important after a hot sweaty session. An ideal meal to consume post training will include carbohydrates and protein. I drink a whey protein shake straight after my early morning strength-training sessions as it's convenient, easy to consume and supports my daily protein requirements.

Post-exercise recovery can be summarised by the 3 Rs: rehydrate, refuel and repair.[42]

- Rehydrate: Replace any water lost through sweating by ensuring you rehydrate with water both during and after exercise. If you have been engaged in a very vigorous and prolonged exercise session, or when you exercise in a hot climate, replacing sodium may also be important. This is because as you sweat you lose salts and minerals, known as electrolytes. Sodium can be obtained via a small salty snack, such as a handful of pretzels, or a vegetable smoothie with a pinch of salt.
- Refuel: A combination of carbohydrates with protein will help replenish glycogen stores and assist with tissue repair.
- Repair: Adequate protein intake assists muscle repair and growth. Consuming protein after an exercise session, as well as a creatine monohydrate supplement, may help enhance recovery. It used to be thought that it was important to consume protein as soon as possible after exercise, but we now know that this isn't necessary. Instead, total protein intake throughout the day is more important than the exact timing.

Supplements for health and sports performance

Whether you need or would benefit from taking supplements will be determined by your lifestyle, health goals and status, and diet. In general, a well-balanced diet can provide you with all the vitamins and minerals you need.

There are a multitude of supplements to choose from that are available to purchase. Many supplements lack robust evidence for their use, however, let's look at four supplements that may be beneficial to consider – vitamin D, omega-3 fatty acids, whey protein and creatine.

Vitamin D
We've already looked at vitamin D on page 93, but here's a reminder that in the UK adults are generally advised to take a vitamin D supplement during the winter months.

Omega-3 fatty acids (fish oil)

If you do not consume two portions of oily fish a week, it is important to consume other foods that contain omega-3, such as nuts and seeds, vegetable oils, and soya or soya products. To ensure you are getting enough omega-3, if you don't eat fatty fish such as salmon, tuna and mackerel, it may be necessary to supplement.

Omega-3 fatty acids play an important function in the body and support healthy ageing, cognitive function, immune response, inflammation and cardiovascular health.

Two omega-3s, eicosapentaenoic acid (EPA) and docosahexaenoic acid (DHA), are found in fatty fish and in omega-3 supplements. A plant-based omega-3, alpha-linolenic acid (ALA), is found in foods such as flaxseeds, chia seeds, walnuts, canola oil and edamame beans.

A high-quality omega-3 supplement will contain at least 80 per cent omega-3 fatty acids, primarily EPA and DHA. If you choose to take an omega-3 supplement, then it's recommended to check the quality by ensuring it's been laboratory-tested and certified by a third party, such as by the International Fish Oil Standards (IFOS) group.[43]

Whey protein

Whey protein is a convenient and easy way to consume protein to meet your daily protein requirements. This can be useful to consume on the go, straight after a workout, as a drink alongside a meal that's low in protein, or when you don't have time for a sit-down meal.

Firstly, let's clarify what whey protein is and where it comes from. When cheese is made from milk, the casein proteins combine to make the cheese. The liquid that is left behind from this process is the whey and contains high-quality protein. Whey is simply a by-product of cheese production and a naturally occurring source of protein. This liquid whey is then dried and turned into whey powder. Whey protein powder comes in a range of flavours and can be mixed with water or milk. I tend to buy vanilla as it tastes pleasant on its own, but it also mixes with other ingredients like berries, flaxseed and oats in smoothies. There are also many plant-based protein powders if you are vegan.

There are numerous research studies that highlight the benefits of protein supplementation with whey protein. One recent study has shown whey protein is more effective for muscle growth in older adults when combined with resistance training than other forms of proteins including meat, casein and soy. This could be due to greater adherence, given that whey protein is relatively easy to consume and cheaper than meat, but regardless of this it remains an important consideration.[44]

Creatine

Creatine is one of the most researched supplements on the market. There are numerous evidence-based benefits of taking this supplement and it's been widely used for many years by both professional athletes and those who exercise regularly. There is now a growing body of evidence to show the benefits of creatine use for women post-menopause for general health and to support the ageing process.

Creatine is a naturally occurring compound that your body produces and stores in your muscle cells and brain, after consuming protein. However, red meat, poultry and fish only contain a small amount of creatine, and you'd need to consume a vast quantity of meat to achieve the same level of creatine in a supplement. Supplementing with creatine helps to increase your phosphocreatine stores and release energy during intense and explosive exercise. It is effective for boosting performance and increasing strength, when combined with resistance training.

There is also growing interest on the effectiveness of creatine for women post-menopause. As well as the sports performance benefits for women who exercise, creatine supplementation appears to have favourable effects on bone strength when combined with resistance training.

Creatine supplementation may also improve our health as we age, as new research continues to emerge showing a wide range of benefits beyond sports performance. Supplementing has been shown to help lower cholesterol and triglyceride levels, reduce fat accumulation in the liver, act as an antioxidant, enhance glycaemic control, increase strength and muscle mass, minimise bone loss, improve functional capacity in people with knee osteoarthritis, have a positive effect on cognitive function and improve mood when combined with an SSRI (selective serotonin reuptake inhibitors) in women with depressive symptoms.[45]

When choosing which creatine supplement to take, creatine mono-hydrate is considered the best and purest option.[46, 47]

CHAPTER 8

YOUR HOME WORKOUT GUIDE

I love going to the gym, as well as training in my personal training studio and my garage, which houses a power rack and Olympic weight plates for my heavier lifting sessions. I find it easier to focus when I am training in a gym, and I benefit from a more extensive range of equipment than I have at home, but I also enjoy riding my bike there and back along the beach.

However much I have always enjoyed the gym environment, I appreciate this isn't for everyone, and as many people discovered during lockdown – it's good to have the option to train in other places.

Not wanting or being unable to go to a gym is a common barrier to exercise. It's why many of my clients have come to me to train in my studio over the years. There are a multitude of reasons why people may not be able to go to a gym or are unwilling to do so. These include lack of childcare, no suitable gym nearby, lack of transport, costs, previous bad experience, and being worried about feeling self-conscious or intimidated. Not having enough spare time is another common barrier to exercise, as it can also be time-consuming to go to a gym, when you consider time spent travelling or waiting for equipment to be free.

The good news is you don't have to go to a gym to enjoy the benefits of physical activity to support healthier ageing. There are many ways to support your health outside of a gym setting, which includes training outdoors, playing a sport, joining a local walking or running group, following online workout videos and exercising at home. You don't need to belong to a gym to do the exercises and workout plans contained in this book, unless you want to. Instead, you'll be able follow them in your own home with minimal equipment. In addition, you may want to utilise an outdoor space for some exercises if you enjoy combining fresh air and exercise at the same time – like I do!

When I'm delivering fitness courses for groups of students, I always start the first day with some general housekeeping points. If you've ever attended a gym induction, you may remember doing something similar. It's essential that exercise is safe and effective, and risks are minimised, which means taking into consideration your environment, the equipment you use, other people in the vicinity, what you wear and your current health status.

With this in mind, let's make your home training experience as safe and effective as possible.

Environment

You don't need a lot of space to exercise, but the space you use must be fit for purpose. Think about which space in your home you would like to exercise in. If it's safe to do so, stand in it, stretch out your arms horizontal to the floor, and turn in a complete circle. If your hands touch anything you need to find a slightly bigger space. Ideally, you need another 10–20 centimetres beyond your fingertips. You may need to consider ceiling height as well – can you reach up or jump up with your arms extended without touching the ceiling?

Now take a good look around the space you intend to exercise in, and complete this checklist.

Exercise environment	Yes	No	Action
Are there any trip hazards, like rugs, clutter, toys or electrical leads?	Yes		Remove rug before each session
Do you need to move smaller items of furniture to create more space when you exercise?			
How well-ventilated is the room, does it have a window you can open, would a fan be helpful in hotter weather?			
Are there any ornaments, a television, a computer or valuable items that could be easily knocked over?			

Exercise environment	Yes	No	Action
Is this space a walkway or thoroughfare where other members of your household walk through frequently?			
Do you have any pets, especially a cat or a dog, and can they be kept out of this space during exercise sessions for their safety and yours?			
Do you have children or grandchildren? If so, can they be kept out of this space when you exercise?			
Is there somewhere suitable in this space where you can put any equipment you will need during your exercise sessions?			
Where is the nearest bathroom? Can you get to it easily enough mid-session if needed?			
Where is the nearest landline, or will you have access to a mobile phone in case of an emergency or accident?			
Where will you get additional water from, if needed, during your session?			

From this list make a note of anything you need to address before you exercise in this space. Although a lot of this might seem like common sense, it's easy to become complacent in our own homes and not see potential dangers.

Exercise is not without risk, but you can minimise the risks to yourself, your surroundings and belongings – and those of others – by doing a thorough and objective assessment before you begin.

Once you are happy that your designated exercise space is free from any potential hazards, I recommend getting into the habit of running through this checklist at the start of each session, and action anything that needs addressing before you begin.

Equipment

The range of exercise equipment available is vast. With so much choice, you may wonder what's best for home use. The good news is that you don't need lots of equipment, or to spend a lot of money for home workouts. With some smart choices you'll be able to complete a range of workouts for the whole body, hitting all the components of fitness we identified at the start of this book. Here's what I recommend.

Equipment essentials	
Exercise mat	A thick padded mat will offer greater comfort for floor exercises, and a non-slip mat is important if you intend to use it on a wood floor or tiles
Two sets of dumbbells	I find most beginners start with a set each of 3kg and 5kg dumbbells. You may need slightly lighter or slightly heavier
Small towel	Useful to wipe equipment down and to mop up sweat
Useful equipment for additional exercises	
Resistance bands with handles	I recommend light, medium and heavy
Short loop resistance bands	Also referred to as glute bands or booty bands
Weighted slam ball	3 or 4kg
Pilates block	
Stopwatch or timer	Alternatively, most mobile phones have a timer you could use

Get in the habit of checking your equipment regularly, wiping it down after use and storing it safely. Weights are best stored at ground level if you don't have a rack designed for this purpose. Be especially vigilant if you have children, grandchildren or pets, to keep them safe from harm.

Your health status

If you've ever worked with a personal trainer or attended a gym or exercise class, you should have filled in a Physical Activity Readiness Questionnaire (PAR-Q). This is part of the initial screening process. Completing a PAR-Q ensures your instructor is aware of your current health status, medical history, pre-existing medical conditions and whether it is safe for you to exercise. In some instances, it may be necessary for a client to have a complete medical evaluation with a doctor before commencing exercise.

There are three possible outcomes from a PAR-Q:

- All clear, no further action required.
- Current health status, medical history or pre-existing medical conditions noted. Modifications and adaptations may be necessary as a result.
- Referral to a medical professional necessary before commencing exercise.

Exercise is not without varying degrees of risk to health, including serious injury and death. Completing a PAR-Q helps minimise these risks and makes the instructor aware of any specific needs the client has. The PAR-Q can also help raise a client's awareness about how their body may respond to exercise.

In the same way, it's important to carry out a self-evaluation on your suitability to exercise, any modifications you might need to make, or whether you need to speak to your doctor before you do the exercises and workouts in this book. Answer yes or no to the following questions.

Physical Activity Readiness Questionnaire (PAR-Q)

	Yes	No
Has your doctor ever said you have a heart condition, and you should only do physical activity recommended by a doctor?		
Have you ever had any form of heart disease?		
Have you ever experienced pain in the chest, neck, jaw, arm or other areas of the body that may indicate lack of blood flow to the heart?		
Do you ever experience shortness of breath at rest or with mild physical exertion?		
Do you lose your balance because of dizziness, or do you ever lose consciousness?		

	Yes	No
Do you have a bone or joint issue that could be made worse from a change in your level of physical activity?		
Are you currently taking any medications for blood pressure or a heart condition?		
Are there any aspects about your health that may be affected by exercise, or that might prohibit your participation?		

If you answered yes to one or more questions:
Talk to your doctor about the questions you answered yes to and seek their advice on whether exercise is suitable for you, or if they recommend any modifications. There could be some exercises they want you to avoid, or they may advise you on restrictions to exercise intensity.

If you answered no to all the questions:
Start slowly and build up gradually. Review how you feel at the end of each exercise session and for the following 24–48 hours. Adjust as necessary for your next session.

Before you exercise always ask yourself, 'how am I feeling today?' This is a good habit to get into and something I ask all my clients at the start of every session. A bad night's sleep, a cold or a sore knee could all indicate you need to modify your session or rest. If you have a temperature, a fever, a chest infection or a gastrointestinal bug, postpone exercise until you feel better.

At all times use your discretion; the PAR-Q doesn't cover every possible medical condition that could increase your risk. If you are in any doubt as to your suitability to exercise, always check with a doctor.

Training principles

Before you begin to exercise, let's consider some basic training principles that will help ensure you get the most from your sessions, work at the right intensity and make progress.

The FITT principle is a useful acronym to remember the components of exercise. FITT stands for frequency, intensity, time and type of exercise. Referring to the FITT principle can help give structure to an exercise plan.

Let's look at how we can apply the FITT principles to the CMO's physical activity guidelines for cardiovascular exercise per week.

'Accumulate 150 minutes of moderate cardiovascular activity (like walking or cycling), or 75 minutes of vigorous cardiovascular intensity (like running) each week, or a combination of the two.'

- F – frequency – not stated*
- I – intensity – moderate or vigorous
- T – time – 150 minutes (moderate) or 75 minutes (vigorous)
- T – type – walking, cycling, or running†

Here's one way to achieve the CMO's recommendation for cardiovascular activity:

- F – frequency – 5 times a week
- I – intensity – moderate
- T – time – 30 minutes
- T – type – walking

Which means five 30-minute walks, each week.

Training principles: cardiovascular exercise

To ensure cardiovascular exercise is safe and effective it's important to achieve the CMO's physical activity guidelines (as a minimum) and to work at an exercise intensity that is appropriate for you.

---

* Determined by how many days you will spread 150 minutes over (or 75 minutes).
† These are just a few suggestions from the CMO as there are many types of cardiovascular activity.

Understanding intensity

In Chapter 1 we looked at heart rate training zones and three different formulas to estimate your maximum heart rate.

To calculate your training zones, work out your percentage HR according to the chart on page 11. If you wear a fitness tracker watch, you'll be able to see your actual heart rate during exercise or look at the data from your watch after your session. You'll then be able to compare this to the training zones.

An alternative way of monitoring exercise intensity is where you rate your level of exertion on a scale 6–20. The Borg scale was developed as a tool to help access physical effort, exertion, breathlessness and fatigue. Each number from 6–20 corresponds to how exercise feels to give a rate of perceived exertion (RPE).[1] The modified Borg scale of 1–10 is more commonly used in fitness settings. Many people find it easier to relate to a scale of 1 to 10 than 6 to 20.

This is a popular and easy way of monitoring exercise intensity that I recommend you use if you are a beginner. Although I wear a fitness tracker watch I still use RPE during my own exercise sessions and when working with clients, as it's quick and simple.

RPE scale (rate of perceived exertion)		
Borg category ratio 1–10 scale	Description	Approximate correspondence to %HRmax
0	Rest	< 57% HRmax
1	Very, very easy	
2	Light activity, easy	57–63% HRmax
3		
4	Moderate to somewhat hard	
5		64–76% HRmax
6		77–95% HRmax
7	Hard to very hard	
8		
9	Extremely hard	96% >HRmax
10	Maximum effort	

Let's bring these numbers to life. Here's how I explain them to my clients:

- 0: At complete rest, sitting in a chair doing nothing at all. You could keep this up all day, it's no effort at all, although boredom might set in!
- 3: Easy, a gentle walking pace that would allow you to walk for an hour, on a level surface, whilst talking to a friend.
- 6: Moderate to somewhat hard, like walking up ten flights of stairs because the lift is broken, and you must keep moving at pace because there's a crowd behind you also climbing the stairs.
- 10: Flat-out sprinting, at maximum effort, like your life depends on it. It's incredibly hard and exhausting, so you can't keep it up for more than a few seconds at a time.

Now you're ready to think about your level of intensity when doing cardiovascular exercise. The cardiovascular workouts in this book include a warm-up, the main cardiovascular session and a cooldown. We will look at warm-ups in closer detail in the next chapter, but for now a warm-up for cardiovascular exercise should gradually elevate the heart rate and the RPE should be 2 rising to 3. A beginner new to cardiovascular training could aim for RPE 4–5 during the main session, whereas intermediate exercisers might achieve RPE 6–8. Regardless of ability, the cooldown should bring everyone back to baseline, which means RPE 3 decreasing to 1.

Once an initial conditioning phase has been achieved – normally over a 6–8-week period – one of the FITT components needs adapting so you can continue to make progress. It's recommended you only alter one component at a time, allow a period of adjustment over another 6–8 weeks before altering another FITT component. In practice this might look like this:

Frequency – increasing cardiovascular sessions from twice weekly to three times a week
Or
Intensity – increasing intensity from RPE 4–5 to RPE 5–6
Or

Time – increasing the duration of your cardiovascular workout
from 20 minutes to 30 minutes
Or
Type – swapping walking for jogging.

Training principles: strength training

To ensure strength training is safe and effective it's important to
achieve the CMO's physical activity guidelines (as a minimum) and
to use a level of resistance that's appropriate for you. This can be
using resistance bands, your body weight, dumbbells or other
weighted training tools – such as a slam ball, power bag or sand
bell.

Strength training involves muscles working against a load or force.
This means a load or force greater than you would normally lift,
carry, pull or push in your day-to-day life. Muscles adapt to this
increased load by getting stronger and bigger, known as muscular
hypertrophy.

How 'heavy' you should lift is determined by your level of experience, training aims and objectives, as well as your health status. It's
recommended that most beginners start with 1–2 sets of 8–12 reps.

A whole-body approach (i.e. training all the main muscle groups)
is important and will support the retention of lean muscle, bone
density and active ageing. In practical terms, this means you should
be able to perform 8–12 reps with good form, but at the end of these
repetitions you are sufficiently fatigued and don't have the strength
to complete further repetitions. This is an important point because if
you can lift a weight for 25 repetitions this will not support gains in
strength and size, although it will support muscular endurance.

Over time, as your muscles adapt to the stimulus of strength training you'll need to overload them in a different way and increase the
difficulty of your session. This is known as the principle of progressive overload.

You can achieve progressive overload in strength training by
changing one of the FITT components.

F – frequency – increase two sessions a week to three
Or
I – intensity – increase the weight
Or
T – time – increase the duration by increasing the number of sets
    or number of exercises, decrease the rest time between sets,
    change the lifting tempo
Or
T – type – change the exercise.

The two sets of dumbbells I have recommended you work with will carry you a long way on this journey. If a weight starts to feel easier, and you can do more than 8–12 reps, you can change one of the other FITT components – such as frequency, time or type of exercise.

In this chapter we've looked at preparing your exercise space, gathering your equipment together and reflecting on your current health status, and I've introduced you to some key training principles alongside the FITT components of fitness. In the next chapter you find a comprehensive range of exercises which will form the basis of the workouts contained in this book to support active ageing.

CHAPTER 9

UNDERSTANDING MOVEMENT

How we move

You probably don't give much thought to how you move as you go about your daily life, although you'll be aware you move in more than one dimension. Take these movements, for example:

- Walking forwards.
- Taking side steps in a narrow space, to get to a seat in a cinema or theatre.
- Turning to look over your shoulder.

Each of these takes place in a different plane of movement. Understanding these planes of movement will help you make sense of why different exercises are beneficial. Ideally, we want our bodies to stay strong and mobile through all the planes of movement, to benefit our function in daily life as well as for any activities we enjoy. For example, twisting movements like a golf swing happen in the transverse plane.

Body movements happen in three different planes of movement, and through different axes. Picture these planes as a flat surface that runs through your body. Each axis is a line at right angles to the plane, about which the body moves.

When you look over your shoulder, from a standing position without moving your feet, this is happening in the transverse plane, and the axis runs through the middle of your body from your feet to the crown of your head. Your torso and neck twist and rotate around this axis in this transverse plane.

This is why we include rotational movements in a warm-up and during the main exercise session. I hope this is a bit of a lightbulb

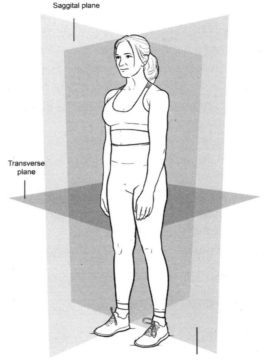

moment for you if you haven't considered this before. Exercise involves body movements; some exercises happen in more than one plane. But I don't want you to see exercise as simply exercise, I really want you to understand how exercise links to the way our bodies are designed to function and move for life.

Sagittal plane – divides body into right and left side. Movement examples: walking, jumping, squatting.

Frontal plane – divides body into front and back. Movement examples: side to side steps, lateral arm or leg raises.

Transverse plane – divides the body horizontally into top and bottom. Movement examples: rotational movements, getting into a car, swimming with breaststroke, hitting a ball in a racket sport.

The workouts in this book incorporate exercises designed to keep you functionally strong in all three planes of movement.

Movement descriptions
- Abduction: Limb moves away from the body, such as lifting an arm out to the side.
- Adduction: Limb moves towards the body, such as squeezing the thighs together.
- Extension: Joint angle increases, such as the elbow joint when the arm is long and extended.
- Flexion: Joint angle decreases, such as bending the knee.
- Internal rotation: Rotating the limb inwards, such as toes turned inwards.
- External rotation: Rotating the limb outwards, such as heels together, toes outwards.
- Dorsi flexion: Point toes towards the face.
- Plantar flexion: Point toes and foot downwards.

Bones, muscles and joints

Your bones, muscles and joints make up your musculoskeletal system.

Bones

Your skeleton is made up of 206 bones. It supports your body, helps you to move and protects your internal organs. Your bones produce blood cells and store and release minerals and fats. Bone is living tissue with the ability to renew and repair from the minute you are born, right into adulthood.

Joints

A joint is where two bones in your body meet and enable movement to occur. Different joints facilitate different types of movement. For example, the knee and elbow are hinge joints which allow flexion and extension. The knee joint is not designed to rotate, which helps explain why a meniscus tear is a common sports injury to the knee caused by rotating and twisting. The meniscus is the cartilage between bones in the knee.

These are the purposes of the various joints in the body:

- Hinge joints: These act like the hinge on a door and allow flexion and extension. The elbow, knee and ankle are hinge joints.
- Ball and socket joints: These allow movement in many directions, including flexion, extension, abduction, adduction, internal and external rotation. The hips and shoulders are ball and socket joints.
- Pivot joint: This allows rotational movement. The neck, between the top two vertebrae, is a pivot joint allowing rotational movement of the head.
- Condyloid joint: This allows flexion and extension as well as side-to-side movement. The wrist is an example of a condyloid joint.

Skeletal muscle

There are more than 600 muscles in your body, made up of skeletal, smooth and cardiac muscle. Skeletal muscles are those involved in voluntary movement. Skeletal muscle attaches to bone, via tendons, to create movement. Muscles work together to allow this movement to happen. They do this through contracting and shortening, and relaxing and lengthening.

How muscles work

The muscles in your body work together to pull on bones and facilitate movement. For example, when you stand up from a chair the muscles in your thighs, calves, bottom, tummy and back are utilised.

Let's look at an everyday activity and how your muscles are working together when you pick up a mug to drink your coffee. As you bring a mug up to your mouth to drink from it, the muscles at the front of your upper arm – your biceps – are contracting and shortening, known as a concentric contraction. The muscles at the back of your upper arm – your triceps – are relaxing and lengthening at the same time.

An eccentric contraction is another way in which muscles work to control and resist movement. This is where a muscle lengthens under tension. A good example of this is how the muscles at the front of your thigh – the quads – lengthen under tension when you walk down a flight of stairs. In this way the movement is controlled as you try to resist the pull of gravity and prevents you falling down the stairs.

Another type of muscle contraction is an isometric contraction, where a muscle or muscles are held in a contracted state but are neither lengthening nor shortening. A plank is a good example of an isometric exercise, where the abdominal muscles are braced but not shortening.

To stay strong and mobile, as an active ager we need to be including exercises that work muscles through the whole range of movement, both contracting and lengthening, as well as loading them eccentrically and isometrically. A well-rounded training programme includes exercises that strengthen all the main muscle groups in the body. Being able to visualise and identify where these muscles are located can help aid mind-muscle connection, bringing attention to specific areas of the body as you move. You may find it helpful to refer to this illustration alongside the exercise descriptions in this book.

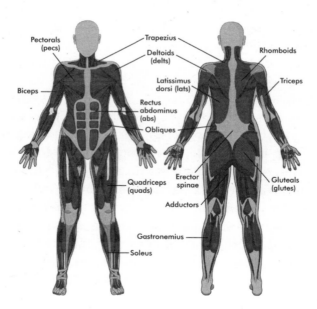

Posture awareness

Posture refers to how your body is positioned when either standing, sitting or lying down. It's important to consider your posture before you begin an exercise programme. This is because how we stand and sit can have a big impact on exercise, our ability to expand our lungs to breathe fully and the risk of injury.

We can further define posture as:

- Static posture: How you hold yourself when standing, sitting or lying down.
- Dynamic posture: How you hold yourself when moving – such as walking, throwing or picking up something.

Several factors influence posture, including gravity, genetics, body type, lifestyle, injury, mental health, muscle length, pregnancy, footwear and age.

The older we are, the longer we have been exposed to gravity and the longer our lifestyle choices may have influenced posture. A previous injury could have led to joint restrictions and compensations elsewhere in the body, which can also affect posture. Depression and stress impact demeanour and posture; downcast means literally looking downwards, which throws the whole body out of alignment. Even what you wear on your feet can make the difference between 'good' and 'bad' posture.

You probably already have an idea of what 'bad' posture looks like, including stooping, slouching, rounded shoulders, head jutting forward and a protruding abdomen. But good posture is more than simply standing up straight.

Posture is better understood if we consider the alignment of the body and what is often referred to as neutral spine. Neutral spine is the natural 'S' shape and position of the spine, which has three curves. These are, from top to bottom, the cervical spine (neck), thoracic spine (middle section) and lumbar spine (lower). In this position the spine acts as a spring to absorb forces, and the limbs, joints, muscles and ligaments are aligned in a way that minimises stress. The body is better balanced in neutral spine and is slower to fatigue.

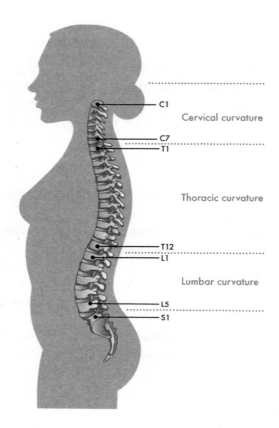

Cervical curvature

Thoracic curvature

Lumbar curvature

Ideal posture will look different for everyone because the precise 'S' curve of your spine is individual to you, so there's no such thing as perfect posture. Your ideal posture will be where your body experiences least resistance. If you have osteoporosis, you may have thoracic kyphosis, with increased curvature in the thoracic area of the spine. Whereas lumbar lordosis, with increased curvature in the lumbar spine, is often seen during pregnancy, or when excess body fat has accumulated around the abdomen.

You don't need to remain in your ideal posture or close to neutral spine all day, though – this is not the aim. Any posture held for an extended period is potentially detrimental. Instead, it's helpful to move throughout the day, check in with posture from time to time, review how you are standing and sitting, and make sure you're not slumped or rounded for extended periods of time.

Find your neutral spine

Try this exercise barefoot, as shoes prevent your toes spreading and may inhibit the distribution of your body weight evenly across your feet, and anything with a heel, or too much cushioning, can throw your pelvis out of alignment and affect your pelvic floor.

1. Stand on a level surface, feet together, and relax your arms at your sides.
2. Turn your toes outwards, followed by your heels, so that your feet end up about hip distance apart. Keep your knees soft.
3. Stretch your toes up, then place them down again, focusing on allowing them to spread out. Feel your body weight spread over the whole area of both feet, front and back.
4. Imagine a thread is pulling you upwards through the crown of your head, helping you to stand tall and lengthen your spine.
5. Allow your eyes to look at the horizon, imagine your chin is resting on a shelf, so that your head is neutral and feels balanced and comfortable at the top of your spine.
6. With an inhale, lift your shoulders upwards, creating a feeling of tension, and as you exhale gently sink your shoulders downwards, imagining your shoulder blades are being placed into a back pocket, and feeling your neck is long and free of tension. It may help to try this a couple of times.
7. Imagine your pelvis is a bowl with a marble at its base. Tilt your pelvis backwards and forwards gently, imagining rolling the marble as it tries to find the midpoint. As you complete this gentle rocking action you should feel your tummy muscles tighten, and your back muscles lengthen, followed by your tummy muscles relaxing and your back muscles tightening. Stop when you find the midpoint.
8. Think about your abdomen as you take a deep breath in through your nose, and let your rib cage expand. Gently exhale through your mouth, and as you do so tighten your abdominal muscles, imagining you are making your waist smaller to squeeze into a tight pair of jeans. Now release your abdominal muscles by about 50 per cent, and a further 20–30 per cent, so

that you are left with a little bit of bracing in your abdominal muscles. The bottom of your rib cage should feel like it's aligned over the top of your hip bones.

9. Finally, carry out a mental inventory of your body. You should feel comfortable and experience minimal tension or stress in any of your muscles and joints in this posture. Now bring your attention to your breath as you gently inhale and exhale for 1–2 minutes.

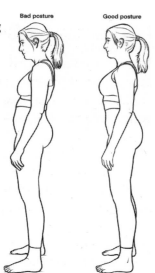

Bad posture　　　　Good posture

The warm-up

Over the years of working and training in gyms, belonging to various running clubs and taking part in fitness events and races, I can confirm that lots of people never warm up before commencing exercise! I regularly see people walk across the gym floor, simply doing a couple of arm swings before heading to the weights. Even when I was delivering fitness courses, I was always astounded at how many people freely confessed to never doing a warm-up.

Perhaps you've been guilty of this too, we have probably all skipped a warm-up at some point. One of the most common reasons people say they do so is a lack of time and a desire to get on with the 'serious' part of the session, and many people simply don't understand the benefits of a warm-up.

But your warm-up deserves to be taken as seriously as the rest of your session, because it's an integral part of the workout. As an active ager it takes on even greater significance. The older we get, the riskier it becomes to skip a warm-up. In the case of an underlying medical condition like high blood pressure, stiff joints and arthritis, diabetes, osteoporosis, obesity or heart disease, an extended and gradual warm-up, over 10–15 minutes, is essential to reduce any exercise associated risk. The older I have grown, the more important my warm-up has become, particularly since experiencing adhesive capsulitis (frozen shoulder) and now having osteoarthritis.

A warm-up helps prepare your body and mind for the work ahead. It aids mobility, joint lubrication, reduces the risk of muscle strain and gently elevates the heart rate. Depending on what type of workout you are going to do, it may also include some specific movement preparation and skill rehearsal – such as body-weight squats before progressing to weighted squats in the main session.

Benefits of a warm-up include:

- Physiological preparation.
- Increased muscle temperature and blood flow.
- Aids joint lubrication.
- Elevates heart rate.
- Psychological preparation.
- Improves performance.

A warm-up also enables you to check in with your body and assess how it's feeling before you commence exercise. It encourages you to take a mental inventory; it's a time when you might notice a little niggle, some joint stiffness, or realise you've slept 'funny' and your neck feels achy. Tuning into how your body is feeling, and doing this every time you exercise, can help you detect when something isn't quite right, or when you feel a little fatigued, as well as when you are full of energy and raring to go.

A good warm-up normally includes a combination of:

- Mobility drills.
- Dynamic active stretching.
- Pulse raising activity.
- Movement or skill rehearsal.

If it's been some time since you've exercised, or you were taught how to warm up several years ago, you may be wondering what's happened to static stretching. Static stretches are where you hold a position in order to stretch a muscle group – no movement is involved, and the stretch is held for 15–30 seconds and up to 2 minutes. Research has shown that static stretching can negatively impact performance, which is why it is no longer recommended at the start of a workout, although it may be beneficial within a warm-up that includes some dynamic movement. Static stretches are still valid and beneficial but are best saved for the end of your session instead.

The specific mobility drills, dynamic stretches, pulse raising activity and skill rehearsals we include in a warm-up will depend on our planned activity. For example, a runner will benefit from focusing on dynamic stretches and movements of the lower limbs, thinking about calves, quads and hamstrings, ankles, knees, hips, feet and Achilles.

Whole-body warm-up activity

This is a general whole-body warm-up with which I recommend you start every exercise session. All the main muscle groups and joints are involved. It incorporates mobility drills, dynamic active stretching, elevates the heart rate and acts as a pulse raiser, and includes some movement and skill rehearsal. It will take you around 5 minutes to complete.

For all these warm-up exercises, start by finding neutral spine, following the instructions on page 145, and make movements slow and controlled, exploring the end of the range of movement available to you. It can help to think about working from the top of your head downwards. Focus on feeling the stretch as the muscles first lengthen and then contract in these movements. Perform 6–8 repetitions of each, more if you notice any stiffness.

Neck and head
1. Gently drop your chin down towards your chest, then tilt it upwards, looking towards the ceiling.
2. Rotate your head to look to the right, then to the left.
3. Drop your right ear towards your left shoulder, then repeat on your right-hand side.

Shoulders
1. Lift your shoulders up to your ears, then roll them backwards and down.

2. Make the movement bigger by circling the arms as you roll the shoulders, extending and raising your arms to the front and up – overhead, backwards and downwards.
3. Reverse the movement by lifting the arms backwards and up overhead, before circling forwards and downwards.
4. Now alternate the arms in a backward crawl, swimming-type movement.
5. Repeat to the front in a front crawl, swimming-type movement.

Chest and upper back

1. Extend your arms on either side of your body, parallel to the floor.
2. With palms facing forwards, bring them across the body in a hug, then open them fully to return to start position.

Abdominals, back and shoulders

1. Widen your stance.
2. Reach your hands upwards and across your body in a diagonal movement to your right, allowing your left heel to lift off the floor as you rotate through your torso, and feel the weight shift to your right leg.
3. Lengthen through your back at the same time so that the arms are outstretched from the top of your fingertips on your right hand, through to the toes on your left foot.
4. Now imagine you are tracing an upside-down rainbow as your hands lead the movement, arcing downwards and then upwards to your left-hand side.
5. As you do this your left heel returns to the floor, so your left foot is balanced and flat, and your right heel lifts upwards as you pivot on the toes of your right foot.
6. Repeat this sweeping arc movement, aiming to rotate a little more with each repetition.

Hips, knees and ankles

1. Continuing with the movement for the abdominals, back and shoulders, now add in a bend in the knees as you try to reach further downwards at the bottom of the arc each time.

Hips

1. Balancing on one leg, lift the other leg to the front, bending at the knee.
2. Circle your knee backwards in a movement that's like opening a door.
3. Bring your forefoot to rest momentarily on the floor after each repetition before repeating.
4. Change legs and perform the same exercise again, this time reversing the movement and lifting the knee to the side, up and forwards like closing a door.
5. Change legs and repeat.

Legs (back of thighs)

1. Swing one leg forwards, pointing your toes towards the ceiling.
2. Reach towards your foot and toes with the opposite arm and hand.
3. Change legs and repeat.

Legs (front of thighs) and knees

1. Bending at the knee, kick your heel upwards and backwards towards your bottom.
2. Change legs and repeat.

Hips, back, legs and bottom

1. Hinge at the hips, pushing your bottom backwards.
2. Keep your knees soft, allow your chest to come towards the floor to act as a counterbalance as you push your hips backwards.
3. Keep your back straight and avoid rounding it.
4. Stretch out your arms so that your torso and arms end up nearly parallel to the floor as your push the hips backwards.

Legs, back, abdominals and shoulders

1. Bend at the knees and sink downwards like you are going to sit on a chair, in a squat movement.

2. At the same time, reach between your knees with your hands, keep your chest up and avoid rounding your back.
3. Straighten up and now reach up over your head, fully extending your body and your arms.

Legs (inner and outer thigh)
1. Take a big step sideways to your right-hand side, bending your right knee. Your left leg should be lengthened and straightened.
2. Sink your hips backwards as you do this and allow your torso to come forwards to act as a counterbalance.
3. Push through your right leg to return to the start position.
4. Repeat on the other side.

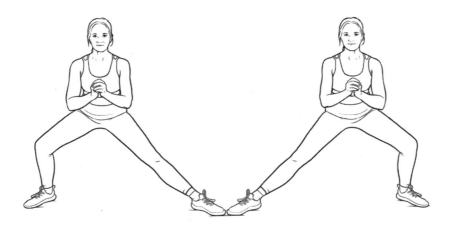

Ankles
1. Keeping your toes on the floor, lift one heel off the floor before gently lowering and lifting your other heel.
2. Pedal your heels alternately, lifting and lowering.

Adaptations and modifications

It's important that you work at a level that's appropriate for you. Here are some ideas on how you can modify the warm-up, if needed, if you want to feel more comfortable or if balance is an issue for you.

1. Sit down on a chair to perform some of these movements, such as the neck and head, shoulders, chest and upper back and ankle warm-up exercises.
2. Use a chair to act as a support in standing exercises to assist balance in movements such as the hip and leg warm-up exercises.
3. Use a chair to act as a support in the hips, back, legs and bottom warm-up exercises.
4. Sit in a chair or have a chair behind you for an added sense of security in the leg, back, abdominals and shoulders warm-up exercises.
5. Sit in a chair or have a chair behind you for an added sense of security in the leg (inner and outer thigh) warm-up exercise.

Additional floor-based dynamic mobility exercises

These additional exercises are a little more advanced. They are not essential to any of the workouts in this book, but if you are able to perform these, they will assist greater mobility.

Perform 6–8 repetitions of each, more if you notice any stiffness.

All fours to downward dog

1. Start from an all-fours position on the floor, resting on your toes and palms of your hands.
2. Push the hips backwards and your heels towards the floor, so that you are inverted and make a triangle shape with the floor.
3. Return to the start position.

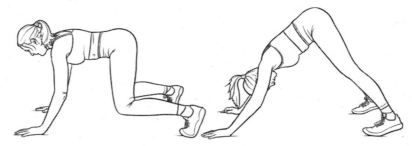

Cat cow

1. Start in an all-fours position.
2. Exhale as you round the spine upwards, tucking the head and pelvis downwards.
3. Inhale, release the back to the start position and continue in a flowing movement, allowing your belly to drop downwards.
4. Lift your head and neck, then tilt your pelvis upwards as your spine curves downwards.

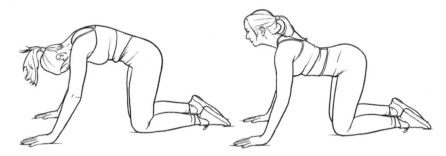

Hand behind head thoracic rotation

1. Start in an all-fours position.
2. Take your right hand and place it on the side of your head.
3. Exhale and rotate your torso by leading the movement with your right elbow upwards.
4. Look towards your elbow.
5. Inhale and return to the start position.
6. Repeat on the other side.

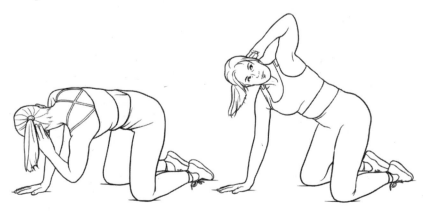

Floor angel

1. Lie on your back, then bend both knees, keeping the feet flat on the floor.
2. Rest your arms on the floor, above your head.
3. Bend your elbows to a right angle and in line with your shoulders, palms up.
4. Slide the elbows down, slightly pressing them into the floor to make a 'V' shape with your body.
5. Now slide your elbows upwards, maintaining a 'V' shape between your upper arm and forearm.
6. Bring your fingertips together above your head as you slide your arms upwards.
7. Slide your elbows downwards again.

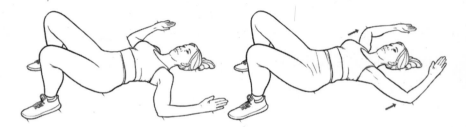

World's greatest stretch

1. Start in a high plank position (page 154).
2. Step your right foot to the outside of your right hand.
3. Pushing your left hand into the ground, lift your right hand and arm, stretching it vertically upwards, rotating through the torso.
4. Return your right hand to the floor, then return your right foot to the start position.
5. Repeat on the other side.

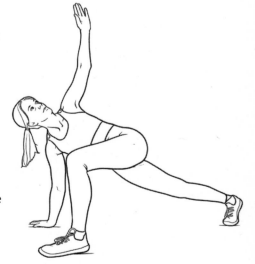

Half-kneeling lunge to hamstring stretch

1. Start in a lunge position (page 169), kneeling on your left knee and extending your right leg, bending at the knee and with your foot on the ground. Both knees should now be at 90 degrees.
2. Push the hips backwards, allowing your right leg to extend, and reach your hands forward towards your right foot.
3. Now reverse the movement, this time lifting your arms up overhead, and pushing your hips further forwards.
4. Repeat on the other side.

Adductor rock back

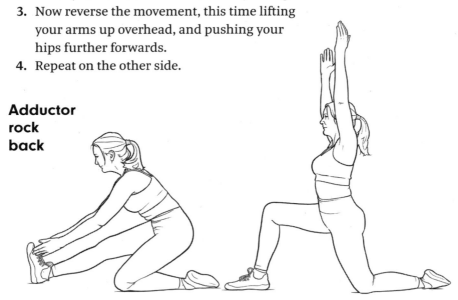

1. From an all-fours position, extend one leg along the floor to the side.
2. Now rock the hips backwards to increase the stretch.
3. Repeat, rocking backwards and forwards.
4. Repeat on the other side.

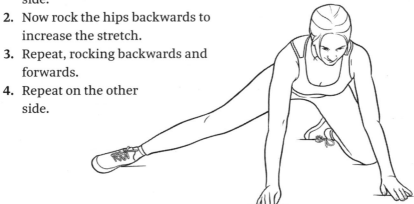

Adaptations and modifications

1. *All fours to downward dog:* Raising yourself from the floor makes this exercise easier. You can either slightly elevate your hands by placing them on Pilates blocks, or higher by resting them on a chair.
2. *Cat cow:* Perform this exercise while seated, with your hands resting on your thighs.
3. *Hand behind head thoracic rotation:* Perform this exercise while seated. Reach and place your left hand on the outside of your right thigh. Cradling your head with your right hand, rotate your torso to your right, leading the movement with your right elbow and looking towards it. Repeat on the other side.
4. *Floor angel:* Perform this exercise while seated on the floor with your back against a wall, or on a chair.
5. *World's greatest stretch:* Use a chair. Place your hands on the seat of the chair and perform the exercise from this elevated hand position.

Cardiovascular exercises

The body-weight exercises in this section create a cardiovascular training effect when repeated multiple times and/or when performed in a circuit with other body-weight exercises or strength exercises. In Chapter 10 you'll see how these individual cardiovascular exercises are combined with others to create dynamic and engaging cardiovascular workouts and circuits working in all three planes of motion. These cardiovascular exercises should always be preceded by the whole-body warm-up on page 148.

Heel-raise walking

1. Stand with feet hip distance apart, with soft knees.
2. Bring one heel up slightly, leaving your forefoot and toes in contact with the floor, to begin heel-raise walking on the spot. Repeat, alternating each leg.

3. As you 'walk', allow your arms to swing naturally – opposite arm to opposite heel raise.

Walking on the spot

1. Lift one knee slightly to begin walking on the spot, but keep your toes in contact with the floor.
2. Lift the whole foot off the floor, then repeat, alternating with the other leg.
3. As you 'walk', allow your arms to swing naturally – opposite arm swings forwards to the raised knee.

Marching on the spot

1. Bring one knee up high to begin marching on the spot.
2. Bend at the elbows, swinging the arms forcefully, opposite arm to high knee.

Fast feet on the spot

1. Stand with your feet slightly wider than hip distance apart, with a small bend in your knees.
2. Alternate lifting your feet off the floor a small distance.
3. Increase the speed until your feet are moving as fast as possible.

Running on the spot

1. Stand with feet hip distance apart, with soft knees.
2. Bend the elbows to about 90 degrees, so the forearms are parallel to the floor.
3. With a slight bend in the knee, kick one foot backwards, then swap to the other in a running motion.
4. At the same time, pump the arms forwards and backwards alternately.

Side toe taps

1. Stand with feet hip distance apart, with soft knees.
2. Bend the elbows to about 90 degrees, so that the forearms are parallel to the floor.
3. Tap your right foot out to the side and back in again quickly, leading the movement with your toes.
4. As you tap your right foot out to the side, bring your right arm forwards in front of you and your left arm backwards, so it is behind you.
5. As you bring your right foot back again, bring your left arm forwards and your right arm backwards.
6. Repeat steps 3 to 5 on other side.

Toe taps to Pilates block

1. Stand with feet hip distance apart, with soft knees.
2. Place a Pilates block flat on the floor, just in front of your feet.
3. Tap the ball and toes of your right foot on the block.
4. Step or hop back, then swap feet.

Lateral lunge with or without touchdown

1. Stand with feet hip distance apart, with soft knees.
2. Step the right foot sideways, bending at the knee, before rapidly driving back to a standing position and stepping to the other side.
3. Add in a touchdown to increase intensity; as you step sideways, reach down to your foot with your opposite hand.

Horizontal rope pulls

1. Stand with your feet set slightly wider than hip distance apart, with soft knees.
2. Stretch your arms out in front of you, parallel to the floor, with a slight bend in the elbow.
3. Imagine you are pulling on a rope with a heavy weight on the end of it; alternate your hands, reaching forwards, making a fist and pulling on the rope.

4. Allow your torso to twist a little with each pull as you rotate and reach to grab the 'rope'.

Vertical rope pulls

1. Stand with your feet set slightly wider than hip distance apart, with soft knees.
2. Stretch and reach your arms up overhead with a slight bend in the elbow.
3. Imagine you are pulling on a bell rope; alternate your hands, reaching upwards, making a fist and pulling on the rope.
4. Allow your upper back to lengthen as you reach to pull the rope on one side and then on the other side.

Rotation with jab

1. Stand with feet slightly wider than hip distance apart, with soft knees.
2. Make a fist with both hands.
3. Bending your elbows, and tucking them in tight to the upper body, bring your fists just under the chin.
4. Rotate to your right, pivoting on your left toe and at the same time jab your left fist, extending your arm across your body to the right-hand side at shoulder height.
5. Return quickly to start position, drawing the extended arm back into the body and the fist under the chin.

Rotation with jab and kick

1. Stand with feet slightly wider than hip distance apart, with soft knees.
2. Make a fist with both hands.
3. Bending your elbows, and tucking them in tight to the upper body, bring your fists just under the chin.
4. Rotate to your right, pivoting on your left toe and at the same time jab your left fist, extending your arm across your body to the right-hand side at shoulder height.
5. Return quickly to start position, drawing the extended arm back into the body and the fist under the chin.
6. Lift the right foot from the floor and, bending at the knee, kick forwards, leading with your heel. At the same time, bring the fists rapidly downwards to either side of the body.
7. Return quickly to start position, drawing the extended arm back into the body and the fist under the chin.

Running arms

1. Stand with feet slightly wider than hip distance apart, with soft knees.
2. Bend the elbows to about 90 degrees, so that the forearms are parallel to the floor.
3. Pump the arms forwards and backwards alternately, allowing the torso to twist from side to side as you do so.

Walkouts

1. Stand with feet hip distance apart, with soft knees, arms hanging at your sides.
2. Push the hips backwards and gently roll your back downwards, extending your arms down towards the ground and your feet.
3. Bend the knees, if necessary, to allow your hands to reach the floor just in front of your feet.
4. Walk your hands forwards until your body makes a line parallel to the ground and you end up in a high plank position.

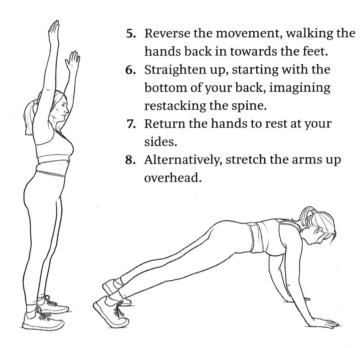

5. Reverse the movement, walking the hands back in towards the feet.
6. Straighten up, starting with the bottom of your back, imagining restacking the spine.
7. Return the hands to rest at your sides.
8. Alternatively, stretch the arms up overhead.

Mountain climbers

1. Start in a high plank position (page 177).
2. Draw one knee up towards the chest before returning to the plank position.
3. Alternate your knees, drawing them up rapidly towards the chest and jumping the foot back each time.
4. Keep your back flat and straight.

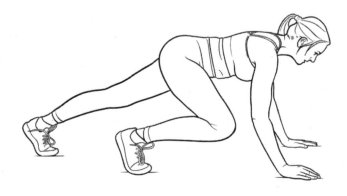

Half jacks

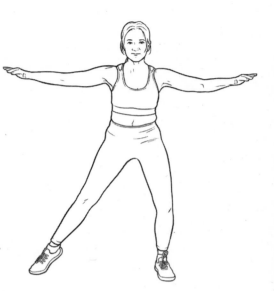

1. Stand with feet hip distance apart, with soft knees, arms hanging at your sides.
2. Step the right leg out to the side, then tap your toes down whilst shifting your body weight to the left leg.
3. At the same time, raise your arms laterally, extending them so they are parallel to the ground.
4. Repeat on the other side.

Jumping jacks

1. Stand with feet together, with soft knees, arms hanging at your sides.
2. Jump the feet outwards on either side.
3. At the same time, raise both arms out sideways in an arc upwards towards your ears.
4. Jump the feet back in and bring the arms back to your sides.

Mock skipping

1. Lightly clasp each hand into a mock fist, as though you are holding a skipping rope.
2. Bending at the elbows, take the hands on either side of your body.
3. Lead small circular movements with your wrists to your elbows, to create a mock skipping action. At the same time, skip your feet alternately or together.
4. Keep your feet close to the ground at first, without jumping, heels slightly raised, landing lightly on the balls of your feet.

Side shuffles or steps

1. Stand with feet hip distance apart, with soft knees.
2. Step to the right-hand side, leading with the right foot.
3. Bring your left foot in to join your right foot.
4. Step to the left-hand side, leading with the left foot.
5. Bring your right foot in to join your left foot.
6. As you speed up, bring the arms into a pumping action, alternating left and right.

Butt kicks

1. Stand with feet hip distance apart, with soft knees.
2. Alternate kicking your heels upwards and backwards towards your bottom.
3. Lightly jump or step from one foot to the other.
4. Alternate the arms in a running motion with the butt kicks.

Skaters with touchdown

1. Stand with feet hip distance apart, with soft knees.
2. Take a wide single leg jump to the right-hand side on your right foot.
3. Bending your left knee, the left foot comes behind your right leg and hovers in mid-air.

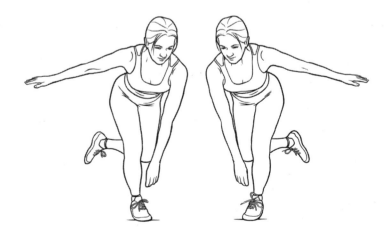

4. Push the hips backwards slightly and touch your left hand down to the floor just in front of your right foot.
5. Repeat on the other side.

Stepping skaters with knee touch

1. Stand with feet hip distance apart, with soft knees.
2. Step to the right-hand side, leading with the right foot.
3. Take the left foot across and behind the right foot in a curtsy movement.
4. Push the hips backwards slightly and touch your left hand to your right knee.
5. Repeat on the other side.

Standing knee drive with arms

1. From a standing position, take a step backwards with your left foot.
2. Bend the right knee.
3. Straighten the left leg.
4. Reach and extend both arms up overhead.

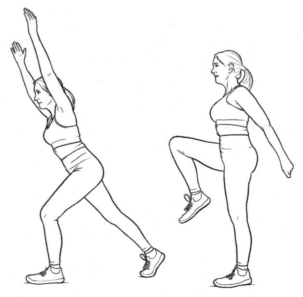

5. Bend and drive the left knee upwards. At the same time, bring the arms and hands down rapidly on either side of the body.
6. Step the left foot back to the start position, reaching and extending both arms up overhead again.
7. Repeat on the other side.

Squat drives

1. Stand with your feet slightly wider than hip distance apart, arms relaxed at your sides.
2. Sit back and down like you are going to sit on a chair. At the same time, lift your arms up in front of you, parallel to the ground.
3. Imagine your feet are glued to the ground, then rapidly drive yourself upwards, out of the squat to the start position. At the same time, drive the arms downwards to your sides.

Squat jumps

1. Stand with your feet slightly wider than hip distance apart, arms relaxed at your sides.
2. Sit back and down like you are going to sit on a chair. At the same time, lift your arms up in front of you, parallel to the ground.

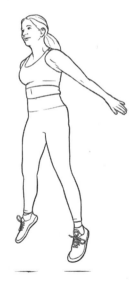

3. Now rapidly drive yourself upwards, into a jump. At the same time, drive the arms downwards and backwards as you jump upwards.

Plank jacks

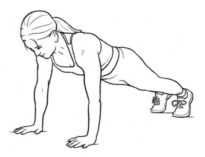

1. Start in a high plank (page 177) or low plank (page 176) position.
2. Jump both feet outwards.
3. Keep the back flat.
4. Jump the feet back in again.

Adaptations and modifications

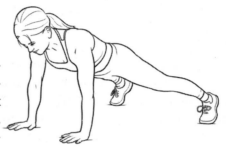

Most of these cardiovascular exercises are performed from a standing position. Many of them work equally well from a seated position. The walkouts and mountain climbers can be modified by placing your hands on a raised surface, like a chair or table.

General principles of strength training and body-weight exercises

Before performing these exercises, let's clarify some general principles.

-   Breathing: Inhaling helps you to prepare and set up for the exercise; try doing this to a count of three. The tempo should be as though you are speaking – and one and two and three. Perform the effort part of the exercise (normally the bit that feels the hardest) by exhaling through pursed lips to another count of three.
-   Bracing core and pelvic floor: As you exhale, think about drawing your rib cage downwards, tightening your abdominal muscles, and lifting your pelvic floor muscles.
-   Neutral spine: Adopt neutral spine unless otherwise stated.

- Grip: When holding the dumbbells use a closed grip, which means the fingers and thumbs are wrapped around the dumbbells, holding them securely.
- Neutral grip: Palms face each other.
- Overhand pronated grip: Palms face downwards.
- Underhand supinated grip: Palms face upwards.

Body-weight strength exercises

Wall push

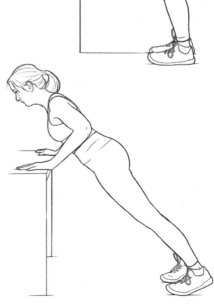

1. Stand facing a wall, feet hip distance apart, so that when you outstretch your arms your hands can reach the wall.
2. Lift and raise your arms slightly wider than shoulder distance apart, parallel to the floor, and place the palms flat on the wall.
3. Keeping your body in a straight line, slowly bend at the elbows, bringing your chest towards the wall.
4. Keep the elbows pointing downwards throughout the movement.
5. Push back to start position.

Countertop push up

1. Stand facing a kitchen worktop or something sturdy of similar height, feet hip distance apart.
2. Stand at a distance so that your hands can reach the worktop.
3. Lift and raise your arms slightly wider than shoulder distance apart, then place your hands on the edge of the worktop.

4. Keeping your body in a straight line, slowly bend at the elbows, bringing your chest towards the worktop.
5. Keep the elbows pointing down and back throughout the movement.
6. Push back to start position.

Modified push ups

1. Start in a high plank position (page 177).
2. Bring your knees down so that your shins and tops of your feet are resting flat on the floor.
3. Lower your torso down towards the floor, keeping your head in line with the spine. Keep the elbows tucked in.
4. Push back to the start position.

Push ups

1. Start in a high plank position (page 177).
2. Lower your body down towards the floor, keeping your head in line with the spine. Keep the elbows tucked in.
3. Push back to the start position.

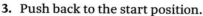

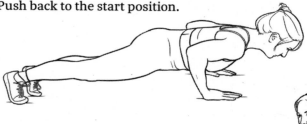

Squats

1. Stand with your feet slightly wider than hip distance apart, arms relaxed at your sides.
2. Sit back and down like you are going to sit on a chair.
3. At the same time, lift your arms up in front of you parallel to the ground, or cross them over your chest.
4. Stand back up again.

Split squats

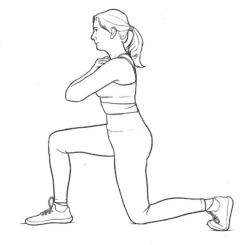

1. From a standing position, feet hip distance apart, step forwards on your right foot so that you are in a staggered stance.
2. Lift your left heel and balance on your forefoot.
3. Lower yourself to the ground, bending both knees. Knees should be bent at a 90-degree angle at the bottom of the movement.
4. Push upwards from this bottom position, back to the staggered stance, extending both knees.
5. Repeat on the other side.

Forward lunge

1. From a standing position, feet hip distance apart, step forwards on your right foot so that you are in a staggered stance.
2. Lift your left heel and balance on your forefoot.
3. Lower yourself to the ground, bending both knees. Knees should be bent at a 90-degree angle at the bottom of the movement.
4. Drive up and backwards, returning your right foot to the start position, alongside your left foot, hip distance apart.
5. Repeat on the other side.

Reverse lunge

1. From a standing position, feet hip distance apart, step backwards on your right foot so that you are in a staggered stance.
2. Balance on the forefoot of your right foot.
3. Lower yourself to the ground, bending both knees. Knees should be bent at a 90-degree angle at the bottom of the movement.

4. Drive up and forwards, returning your right foot to the start position, alongside your left foot, hip distance apart.
5. Repeat on the other side.

Lateral lunge

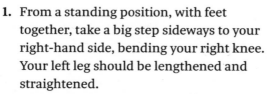

1. From a standing position, with feet together, take a big step sideways to your right-hand side, bending your right knee. Your left leg should be lengthened and straightened.
2. Sink your hips backwards as you do this and allow your torso to come forwards to act as a counterbalance.
3. Push through your right leg to return to the start position.
4. Repeat on the other side.

Floor dips

1. Sit on the floor and extend your legs to the front, bending at the knee.
2. Lean backwards slightly.
3. Rest your hands, with fingers pointing forwards, on the floor on either side of your body.
4. Keeping the elbows close to the body, push yourself upwards, raising your hips off the floor.
5. Lower downwards without letting your bottom touch the floor.

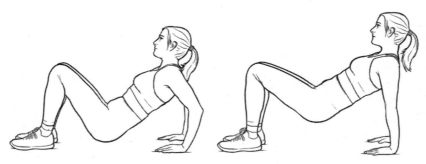

Adaptations and modifications

Body-weight strength exercises are mostly modified by reducing the range of movement performed. In the lateral lunge, for example, you could take a smaller step to the side; in the squat, you could reduce the depth by performing a semi-squat.

Core body-weight exercises

The following exercises focus on building strength in the core, which includes your abdominal muscles and back muscles.

Pelvic tilt

1. Lie on your back, legs extended with knees bent and feet flat on the floor.
2. Rest your arms on the floor on either side of your body.
3. Inhale through your nose.
4. As you exhale, draw in your tummy muscles, bringing your rib cage down towards your pelvis and flatten your lower back into the floor.
5. Slightly lift your tailbone as your tummy muscles tighten, so that your pelvis is tilted upwards.
6. Inhale as you return to the start position.

Abdominal hollowing

1. Start in an all-fours position, adopting a neutral spine, with the head in line with the spine.
2. Without arching or rounding your back, take a deep breath in through your nose, allowing your abdominal muscles to relax.
3. Exhale through your mouth, and at the same time draw in your abdominal muscles, lifting your belly button upwards.
4. Inhale and repeat.
5. Your back should remain in neutral alignment throughout.

Ab curl

1. Lie on your back, legs extended with knees bent and feet flat on the floor.
2. Rest the palms of your hands on your thighs.
3. Inhale through your nose.
4. As you exhale, squeeze your tummy muscles and lift your head and shoulders off the floor. Allow your hands to travel upwards on your thighs as you lift your head and shoulders.
5. Inhale as you lower yourself to the floor again.

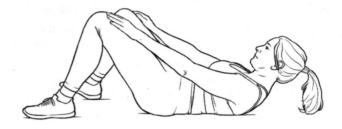

Back extension

1. Lie face down on the floor.
2. Bending at the elbows, rest your forearms on the floor, palms flat on either side of your body.
3. Inhale through your nose.
4. Exhale through your mouth and at the same time lift your head, back and arms off the floor.
5. Inhale as you return to the start position.

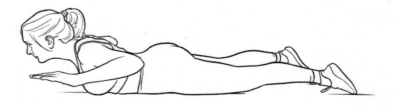

Supine bridge

1. Lie on your back, legs extended with knees bent and feet flat on the floor.
2. Rest your arms on the floor on either side of your body.
3. Inhale through your nose.
4. As you exhale, draw in your tummy muscles, bringing your rib cage down towards your pelvis, and flatten your lower back into the floor.
5. Lift your tailbone as your tummy muscles tighten, so that your pelvis is tilted upwards.
6. Continue to peel your spine off the floor from its base up to your shoulders, so that you end up with your hips elevated off the floor.
7. As you inhale, reverse the movement, starting with the top of your spine as you return to the start position.

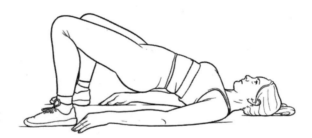

Supine heel taps

1. Lie on your back, legs extended with knees bent and feet flat on the floor.
2. Rest your arms on the floor on either side of your body.
3. Inhale through your nose and raise your right leg. Maintain the knee bend, so that your shin is parallel to the floor, with your knee over your hip. This is referred to as table-top position.

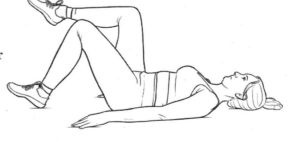

4. As you exhale, take your leg downwards again until your heel lightly touches the floor.
5. Inhale and raise back up again.
6. Repeat on the other side.

Alternate supine heel taps

1. Lie on your back, legs extended with knees bent and feet flat on the floor.
2. Rest your arms on the floor on either side of your body.
3. Inhale through your nose and raise your right leg, maintaining the knee bend, up to a table-top position. Your shin should be parallel to the floor, your knee over your hip.
4. Exhale, and as you inhale again bring your left leg up to join your right in a table-top position.
5. As you exhale take your right leg downwards again until your heel lightly touches the floor.
6. Inhale and raise back up again.
7. Repeat with your left leg.

Dead bug

1. Lie on your back, legs extended with knees bent and feet flat on the floor.
2. Extend your arms upwards so that your elbows and wrists are in alignment with your shoulders.
3. Inhale through your nose and raise your right leg, maintaining the knee bend, up to a table-top position. Your shin should be parallel to the floor, your knee over your hip.

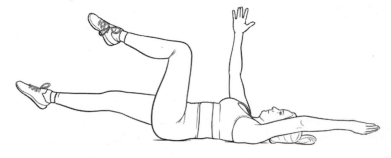

4. Exhale, and as you inhale again bring your left leg up to join your right in a table-top position.
5. As you exhale, extend the right leg outwards parallel to the floor, and at the same time lower your left arm towards the floor.
6. Inhale and return both limbs to the start position.
7. Exhale and repeat with the left leg and right arm.

Bird dog

1. Start in an all-fours position, adopting a neutral spine and with your head in line with the spine.
2. Without arching or rounding your back, take a deep breath in through your nose, allowing your abdominal muscles to relax.
3. Exhale through your mouth and at the same time draw in your abdominal muscles, lifting your belly button upwards, and extend your right arm and left leg outwards so that they are parallel to the ground.
4. Inhale and return both limbs to the start position.
5. Exhale and repeat with left arm and right leg.

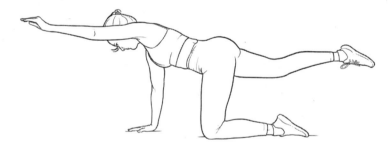

Low plank – kneeling

1. Lie face down on the floor.
2. Bending at the elbows, rest your forearms on the floor, palms flat on either side of your body.
3. Keeping your knees and shins in contact with the floor, push yourself up and slightly backwards onto your forearms. With your shoulders stacked over your elbows, and your head and spine in alignment, this is the low plank kneeling position.

4. Hold this position for 10 seconds initially and up to 30 seconds as you get stronger.

Low plank

1. Lie face down on the floor.
2. Bending at the elbows, rest your forearms on the floor, palms flat on either side of your body.
3. Push yourself up and slightly backwards onto your forearms and onto your toes.
4. With your shoulders stacked over your elbows, and your head and spine in alignment, this is the low plank position.
5. Hold this position for 10 seconds initially and up to 30 seconds as you get stronger.

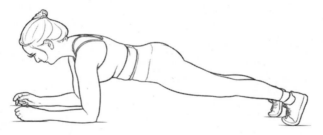

High plank – kneeling

1. Lie face down on the floor.
2. Bending at the elbows, rest your forearms on the floor, palms flat on either side of your body.
3. Keeping your knees and shins in contact with the floor, push yourself up, extending your arms so that you rest on your hands.
4. With your shoulders stacked over your hands and your head and spine in alignment, this is the high plank kneeling position.
5. Hold this position for 10 seconds initially and up to 30 seconds as you get stronger.

High plank

1. Lie face down on the floor.
2. Bending at the elbows, rest your forearms on the floor, palms flat on either side of your body.
3. Push yourself up, extending your arms and rising onto your toes.
4. With your shoulders stacked over your hands and your head and spine in alignment, this is the high plank position.
5. Hold this position for 10 seconds initially and up to 30 seconds as you get stronger.

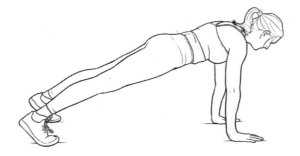

Plank to knee tap

1. From the high plank position, lift your right hand whilst pushing your hips up and backwards.
2. Reach your right hand towards your left knee.
3. Tap your knee with your hand and return to the high plank position.
4. Repeat on the other side.

Plank to foot tap

1. From the high plank position, lift your right hand whilst pushing your hips up and backwards.
2. Reach your right hand towards your left foot.

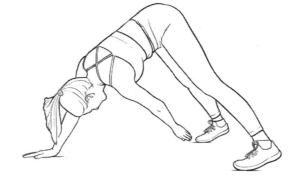

3. Tap your foot with your hand and return to the high plank position.
4. Repeat on the other side.

Half get-up

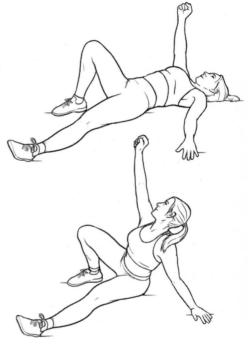

1. Lie on your back.
2. Bend your right knee and rest your right foot on the floor.
3. Extend your right arm upwards, so that your elbow and wrist are in alignment with your shoulder.
4. Extend your left arm out to the side, making a right angle with your body, palm down.
5. Pushing your right foot into the floor, lift your right shoulder and arm off the floor.
6. Shift your weight onto your left forearm before pushing further upwards onto your left hand.
7. You should be seated now in a half get-up position, left leg extended, right knee bent, right arm vertical to the floor with the left arm fully extended with palm flat on the ground.
8. Reverse the movement, sliding down onto your left forearm first, then all the way back down.
9. Ease the rest of the way back to the start position.
10. Repeat on the other side.

Get-up

1. Lie on your back.
2. Bend your right knee, rest your right foot on the floor.
3. Extend your right arm upwards, so that your elbow and wrist are in alignment with your shoulder.

4. Extend your left arm out to the side, making a right angle with your body, palm down.
5. Pushing your right foot into the floor, lift your right shoulder and arm off the floor.
6. Shift your weight onto your left forearm before pushing further upwards onto your left hand.
7. Push your hips upwards so that your weight is split between your right foot and left hand.
8. Bending your left knee, bring your left leg underneath your hips until your left shin can rest on the floor.
9. Push off the floor with your left hand so that you are in a kneeling lunge position with your right arm vertical to the floor.
10. Using your legs, push upwards to a staggered stance before bringing your feet together, hip distance apart.
11. Reverse the sequence to bring yourself back to lying on your back again.

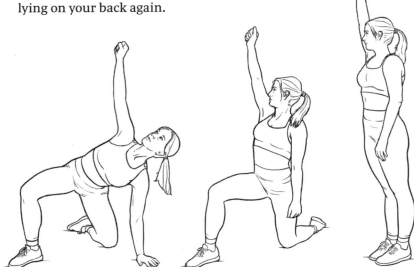

Crab toe reach

1. Sit on the floor, extend your legs to the front, bending at the knee. Lean backwards slightly.
2. Rest your hands, with fingers pointing outwards, on the floor on either side of your body.

3. Keeping the elbows close to the body, push yourself upwards, raising your hips off the floor.
4. Lift and extend your left leg in front of you.
5. Lift and reach towards your left foot with your right hand.
6. Replace your foot and hand back to the floor and repeat on the other side.

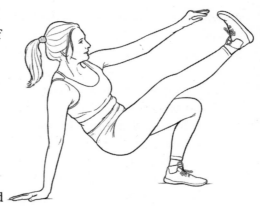

Dumbbell strength exercises

The following strength exercises are performed using either a set of dumbbells or a single one.

A deadlift exercise is a fundamental human movement pattern that involves a hip hinge. Understanding how to perform a deadlift has carryover benefits to daily life and can help you avoid injuring your back. Picking up a delivery box from the floor, lifting a bag of shopping, or bending down to pick up a small child are all examples of where mastering a hip hinge movement and the deadlift can be used effectively.

However, if you have a pre-existing back injury or pain it may be advisable to avoid the following deadlift variations. Instead, work on the core-conditioning exercises in this book to help strengthen your back and abdominal muscles.

Deadlift

1. Place the dumbbells on the floor just to the sides of your feet.
2. Stand with feet hip distance apart.
3. Push your hips backwards and bend at the knees.
4. Keep your chest up, your back straight, with your arms hanging at your sides.

5. Pick up the dumbbells with a closed neutral grip.
6. Keep the dumbbells close to the sides of your body as you slowly straighten your legs and extend your back to return to a standing position.
7. Reverse the movement, pushing your hips backwards and bending at the knees.
8. Keep your chest up, your back straight, with your arms hanging at your sides.
9. Lower the dumbbells as low as your flexibility allows, without rounding your back.
10. Keep the dumbbells close to your body as you slowly drive your hips forwards, straighten your legs, and extend your back to return to a standing position.

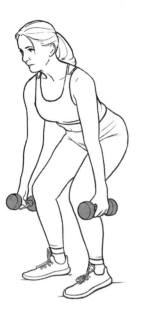

Romanian deadlift

1. Stand with feet hip distance apart.
2. Hold the dumbbells in front of your thighs.
3. Push your hips backwards and bend at the knees.
4. Keep your chest up, your back straight, with arms and dumbbells in front of your body.
5. Lower the dumbbells to mid shin.
6. Keep the dumbbells close to your thighs as you slowly drive your hips forwards, straighten your legs, and extend your back to return to a standing position.

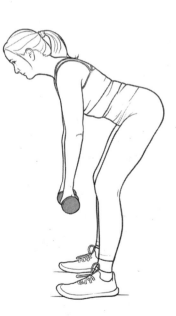

B stance deadlift

1. Hold the dumbbells with a closed neutral grip on either side of your body.
2. Stand with feet hip distance apart, then take your right foot backwards to rest on the ball of your foot.
3. Keeping your left leg straight, push your hips backwards, bending your right knee.
4. Keep your weight on your left leg and use your right foot to stabilise and balance you.
5. Keep your chest up, your back straight, with arms and dumbbells either side of your body.
6. Lower the dumbbells until you feel a stretch in your left leg.
7. Slowly drive your hips forwards and extend your back to return to the start position.
8. Repeat on the other side.

Single leg deadlift

1. Hold the dumbbells in front of your thighs.
2. Lift, raise and straighten your right leg to the back.
3. Balance on your left foot and keep a slight bend in your left knee.
4. Keeping your back flat, allow the dumbbells to slowly travel downwards.
5. Aim for your back and leg to end up parallel with the floor, with your arms and dumbbells at right angles to your body.

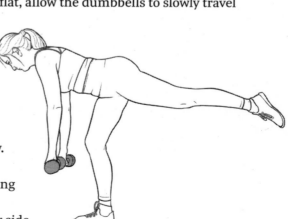

6. Return to the start position by squeezing the glutes.
7. Repeat on the other side.

Goblet squats

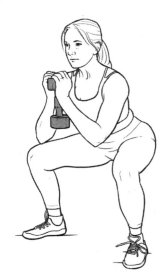

1. Stand with your feet slightly wider than hip distance apart.
2. Hold one dumbbell vertically, gripping it with both hands underneath the wide end of the weight.
3. Bending at your elbows, hold the dumbbell close to your upper body.
4. Slowly sit back and down like you are going to sit on a chair. Keep your chest up.
5. Stand up again.

Split squats

1. Hold the dumbbells on either side of your body, with your arms extended.
2. From a standing position, feet hip distance apart, step forward on your right foot so that you are in a staggered stance.
3. Lift your left heel and balance on your forefoot.
4. Lower yourself to the ground, bending both knees. Knees should be bent at a 90-degree angle at the bottom of the movement.
5. Push upwards from this bottom position, back to the staggered stance, extending both knees.
6. Repeat on the other side.

Forward lunge

1. Hold the dumbbells on either side of your body, with your arms extended.
2. From a standing position, feet hip distance apart, step forward on your right foot so that you are in a staggered stance.
3. Lift your left heel and balance on your forefoot.
4. Lower yourself to the ground, bending both knees. Knees should be bent at a 90-degree angle at the bottom of the movement.

5. Drive up and backwards, returning your right foot to the start position, alongside your left foot, feet hip distance apart.
6. Repeat on the other side.

Reverse lunge

1. Hold the dumbbells on either side of your body, with your arms extended.
2. From a standing position, feet hip distance apart, step backwards on your right foot so that you are in a staggered stance.
3. Balance on the forefoot of your right foot.
4. Lower yourself to the ground, bending both knees. Knees should be bent at a 90-degree angle at the bottom of the movement.
5. Drive up and forwards, returning your right foot to the start position, alongside your left foot, feet hip distance apart.
6. Repeat on the other side.

Lateral lunge

1. Hold the dumbbells on either side of your body, with your arms extended.
2. From a standing position, with feet together, take a big step sideways to your right-hand side, bending your right knee. Your left leg should be lengthened and straightened.
3. Sink your hips backwards as you do this and allow your torso to come forwards and the dumbbells to extend closer to the ground.
4. Push through your right leg to return to the start position.
5. Repeat on the other side.

Chest press

1. Lie on your back, legs extended with knees bent and feet flat on the floor.
2. Take your upper arms away and perpendicular to your body, just below shoulder height.

3. Forearms should be perpendicular to the floor, dumbbells in each hand, palms facing your feet.
4. Press the dumbbells upwards until your arms are almost fully extended. At the top, the dumbbells should be over the mid chest.
5. Slowly return to the start position.

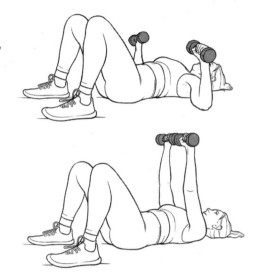

Single arm row

1. Stand with feet hip distance apart, holding a dumbbell in your right hand.
2. Step back on your right leg and bend the left knee at the same time.
3. Your upper body and left leg should be in line with one another and at a 45-degree angle to the floor.
4. Rest your left hand on your left thigh to stabilise your back.
5. The dumbbell in your right hand should be perpendicular to the floor, with your shoulder, elbow and wrist in alignment.

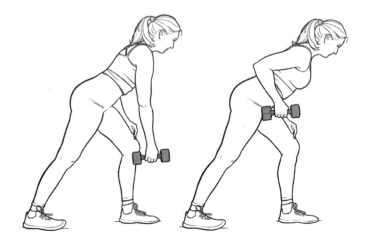

6. Keeping your palm facing your body, and your elbow close to your body, lift the dumbbell towards your waist in a row movement.
7. Slowly return to the start position.
8. Repeat on the other side.

Bent-over row

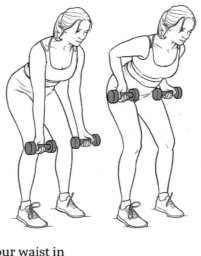

1. Hold the dumbbells on either side of your body with a closed neutral grip.
2. Push the hips back, bending at the knees, keeping your arms perpendicular to the floor. Your back should end up at around a 45-degree angle to the floor.
3. Rotate your shoulders backwards, along with your arms, so your palms face away from your body.
4. Keeping your elbows close to your body, lift the dumbbells towards your waist in a row movement.
5. Slowly return to the start position.

Biceps curls

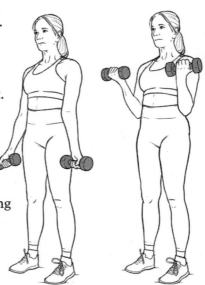

1. Stand with feet hip distance apart.
2. Hold a dumbbell in each hand in front of your thighs, palms facing away from your body.
3. Keeping your upper arms glued to the sides of your body, bend at the elbows and slowly bring the dumbbells up towards your chest.
4. Slowly lower and return to the start position.

Single arm triceps kickback

1. Stand with feet hip distance apart, holding a dumbbell in your right hand.
2. Step back on your right leg and bend the left knee at the same time. Your upper body and left leg should be in line with one another at a 45-degree angle to the floor. Rest your left hand on your left thigh to stabilise your back.
3. The dumbbell in your right hand should be perpendicular to the floor, your shoulder, elbow and wrist in alignment.
4. Draw your right elbow up and keep your upper arm glued to the side of your body.
5. Extend and straighten your arm backwards.
6. Slowly bend at the elbow again and return to the start position.
7. Repeat on the other side.

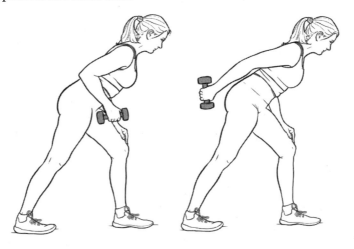

Triceps kickbacks

1. Hold the dumbbells on either side of your body with a closed neutral grip.
2. Push the hips back, bending at the knees, with your arms perpendicular to the floor. Your back should end up at around a 45-degree angle to the floor.

3. Draw both elbows back, keeping your upper arms glued to the sides of your body.
4. Extend and straighten your arms backwards.
5. Slowly bend at the elbows again and return to the start position.

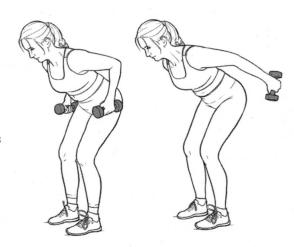

Triceps dips

1. Use a sturdy chair or bench and sit on the edge of it, then place your hands on either side of your bottom, palms flat, fingers facing forwards.
2. With your knees bent at 90 degrees, push your body up and slightly forwards, extending your arms.
3. Slowly bend at the elbows as you lower your bottom towards the floor, keeping your upper body perpendicular to the floor.
4. When you have reached a depth that you can comfortably achieve, use your arms to push back to the start position.

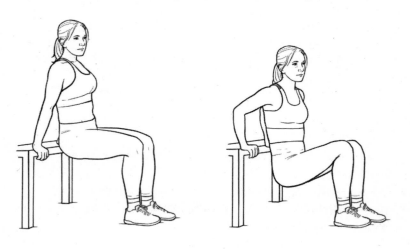

A progression of this exercise is to extend and lengthen your legs with your heels resting on the floor.

Shoulder press

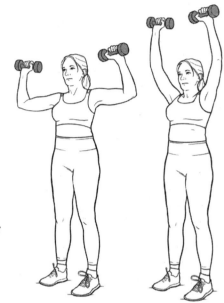

1. Stand with your feet hip distance apart.
2. Hold a dumbbell in each hand with a closed neutral grip. Raise the dumbbells up to shoulder height, or in line with the ears, with your elbows bent. The wrists should be over the elbows.
3. Press the dumbbells up overhead so that wrist, elbow and shoulder are in alignment.
4. Return to the start position.

Lateral raise

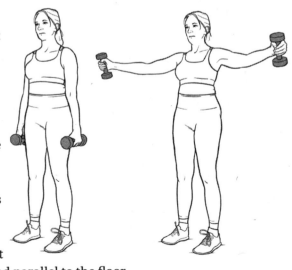

1. Stand with your feet hip distance apart.
2. Hold a dumbbell in each hand with a closed neutral grip, then lift and extend your arms out to the sides, palms facing forwards.
3. Raise the dumbbells on either side, with a light bend in your elbows, to the height of your shoulders and parallel to the floor.
4. Return to the start position.

Alternate front raise

1. Stand with your feet hip distance apart.
2. Hold a dumbbell in each hand with a closed neutral grip, then lift your right arm forwards, palm facing inwards.
3. Raise the dumbbell to the height of your shoulder and parallel to the floor.
4. Return to the start position and repeat on the other side.

Reverse fly

1. Hold the dumbbells with a closed neutral grip on either side of your body.
2. Push the hips back, bending at the knees, with arms perpendicular to the floor. Your back should end up at around a 45-degree angle to the floor.
3. Lift and extend your arms out to the sides, palms facing the floor.
4. Raise the dumbbells on either side, with a slight bend in your elbows, to the height of your shoulders and parallel to the floor.
5. Return to the start position.

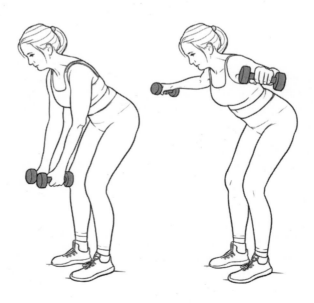

Clean and press

1. Stand with feet hip distance apart, with one dumbbell on the floor near to your feet.
2. Use a squat movement to lower yourself towards the ground so you can pick up the dumbbell in your right hand.
3. As you stand up again, bring the dumbbell up to shoulder height with a bent elbow. The wrist should be over the elbow.
4. Press the dumbbell up overhead so that wrist, elbow and shoulder are in alignment.
5. Return the dumbbell to shoulder height before returning it to the floor again and the start position.
6. Repeat on the other side.

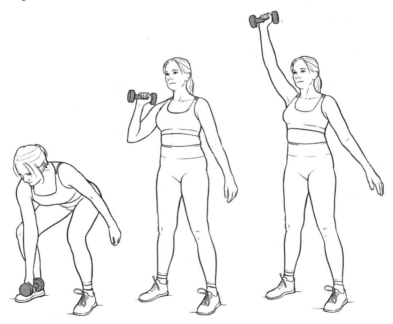

Adaptations and modifications

Dumbbell strength exercises can often be modified by reducing the range of movement, such as placing dumbbells onto a low bench or step to perform deadlifts, by using a chair as support – holding onto one when performing a split squat – and sometimes by swapping to a different exercise that targets the same area of the body, such as a triceps dip instead of a triceps kickback.

Resistance band strength exercises

A resistance band can be a substitute for weights, which works by increasing the tension in the band as it is stretched. Bands come in differing levels of resistance – from light through to very hard or heavy. At the start of each exercise the band needs to be under some tension, with no slackness in it. As the exercise is performed, the tension in the band increases until it is either stretched to its end point or you have reached the end of your range of movement.

An anchor point is needed for some exercises. A body part can act as an anchor point, such as your feet when you stand on the band. A sturdy object such as a stair banister, heavy chair leg or door handle can also act as an anchor point. It's important to check any anchor point is strong enough to withstand you pulling or pushing the band, in order to avoid injury. Another person may also act as an anchor point; this is something I do with clients by holding the middle of the band as the client performs an exercise. If you have a willing partner this might be an option for you too!

Deadlift

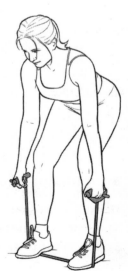

1. Anchor the band under your feet, holding the ends in each hand.
2. Position your feet hip distance apart.
3. Push your hips backwards and bend at the knees.
4. Keep your chest up and your back straight, with your arms hanging at your sides.
5. Make sure the band is under tension at this point with no slackness, then slowly straighten your legs and extend your back to bring yourself to a standing position as the tension in the band increases.

Squats

1. Anchor the band under your feet, holding the ends in each hand.
2. Position your feet hip distance apart.
3. With your arms at your sides, make sure the band is under maximum tension at this point with no slackness, then slowly sit back and down like you are going to sit on a chair. Keep your chest up as you do so.
4. Stand back up again.

Split squats

1. From a standing position, feet hip distance apart, step forwards onto your right foot so that you are in a staggered stance.
2. Anchor the band under your right foot and, holding the ends in each hand, arms at your sides, make sure the band is under maximum tension with no slackness.
3. Lift your left heel and balance on your forefoot.
4. Lower yourself to the ground, bending both knees. Your knees should be bent at a 90-degree angle at the bottom of the movement.
5. Push upwards from this bottom position, back to the staggered stance, extending both knees.
6. Repeat on the other side.

Chest press

1. Lie on your back and place the resistance band underneath your shoulders, holding the ends in each hand.
2. Extend your legs with the knees bent and your feet flat on the floor.
3. Move your upper arms away until perpendicular to your body, just below shoulder height. The forearms should be perpendicular to the floor and the resistance band should be under tension with no slack.
4. Push upwards until your arms are almost fully extended.

5. At the top, the ends of the resistance band should be over the middle of your chest.
6. Slowly return to the start position.

Seated row

1. Sit upright on the floor, with your legs extended but with a slight bend in the knee, feet flexed and toes pointing upwards.
2. Place the resistance band behind the soles of your feet and hold the ends with your palms facing inwards.
3. Extend your arms, ensuring the band is under tension at this point with no slack.
4. Draw the ends of the band towards your waist, keeping your elbows tucked in.
5. Slowly return to the start position.

Biceps curls

1. From a standing position, place the resistance band underneath your feet, holding the ends in each hand with your arms at your sides, palms facing forwards. Ensure the band is under tension at this point, with no slack.
2. Keeping your upper arms glued to the sides of your body, bend at the elbows and slowly bring the ends of the band up towards your chest.
3. Slowly lower and return to the start position.

Single arm triceps extension

1. From a standing position, take hold of one end of the resistance band with your right hand.
2. Extend your arm up overhead, then bend at the elbow so that the length of the resistance band is vertically behind you.
3. Trap the other end of the band or handle underneath your right foot. Ensure the band is under tension at this point with no slack.
4. Keeping your elbow above and in line with your shoulder, extend your arm upwards.
5. Slowly lower and return to the start position.
6. Change sides and repeat.

Lateral raise

1. From a standing position, place the resistance band underneath your feet, holding the ends in each hand, with your arms at your sides, palms facing your body. Ensure the band is under tension at this point with no slack.
2. Lift and extend your arms to the sides, up to the height of your shoulders, parallel to the floor.
3. Slowly lower and return to the start position.

Front raise

1. From a standing position, place the resistance band underneath your feet, holding the ends in each hand, with your arms at your sides, palms facing your body. Ensure the band is under tension at this point with no slack.
2. Lift both your arms to the front, palms facing downwards and raise them to the height of your shoulders, parallel to the floor.
3. Slowly lower and return to the start position.

Pulldown

1. From a standing
position, hold onto the
resistance band,
wrapping each end
around each of your
palms until your
hands are slightly
wider than shoulder
distance apart.
2. Extend your arms up
overhead, vertically.
3. Pull each end of the
band in an arc on
either side of your
body so that your
arms are parallel to the floor and in line with your shoulders.
4. Return to the start position.

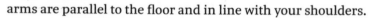

Pull apart

1. From a standing
position, hold onto
the resistance
band, wrapping
each end around
each of your palms
until your hands
are slightly wider
than shoulder
distance apart.
2. Extend and lift
your arms upwards
to shoulder height,
palms facing each other.

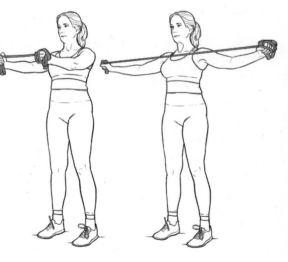

3. Pull the band apart and your palms away from one another until your arms are fully extended on either side of your body in a 'T' shape.
4. Return to the start position.

Y T A

1. Holding each end of the resistance band in each hand, anchor the middle of the band at mid-chest height, then face the anchor point and step backwards.
2. Extend and lift your arms upwards to shoulder height, palms facing each other. This is your start position.
3. Keeping your arms extended, with thumbs and handles rotated away from the body, lift them overhead and outwards at an angle into a 'Y' shape.
4. Return to the start position before lowering your extended arms to the sides of your body in a 'T' shape.
5. Return to the start position before extending your arms and lowering them outwards at an angle into an 'A' shape.
6. Return to the start position.

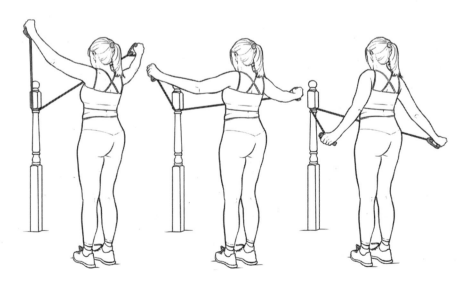

Slam ball exercises

Slam balls are designed to be able to withstand being slammed to the ground or wall without breaking. Used in a gym they are unlikely to do damage to the surroundings, however, you will have to assess the suitability of using a slam ball in your home. In general, I would not recommend using these inside; I use mine outdoors, on grass or hard surfaces that won't break or get damaged.

Overhead slam

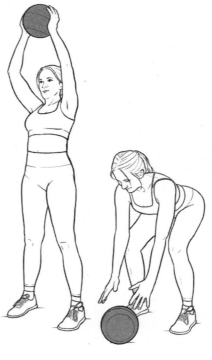

1. Place the slam ball on the ground just in front of your feet.
2. From a standing position, feet hip distance apart, squat down and pick up the slam ball.
3. As you rise up, lift the slam ball overhead with your arms fully extended, then
4. explosively throw the ball downwards to slam on the ground.
5. Pick the ball up and repeat.

Rainbow slam

1. Place the slam ball on the ground to the left of your feet.
2. From a standing position, feet hip distance apart, bend at the knees to reach down sideways and pick up the slam ball.
3. Rise and lift the slam ball up overhead, rotating slightly to your right with arms fully extended, then explosively throw the ball downwards to slam on the ground to the right of your feet.
4. Pick the ball up and repeat on the other side so that each time the slam ball is being lifted overhead in an arc like a rainbow.

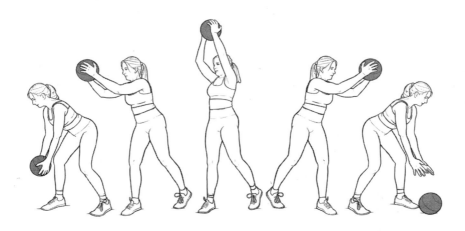

Squat throw

1. Stand with feet hip distance apart and hold the slam ball at chest height.
2. Lower yourself into a squat, then explosively drive back to a standing position whilst throwing the slam ball upwards.
3. Either catch the ball on the way down to repeat again, or take a small step backwards and allow the ball to hit the ground before picking up again and repeating.

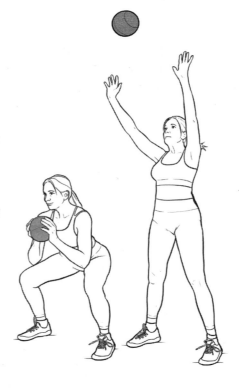

Squat to wall ball slam

1. Stand facing a wall, arm's length away, with feet hip distance apart and holding the slam ball at chest height.
2. Lower into a squat, then explosively drive back to a standing position whilst throwing the slam ball upwards against the wall.
3. Catch the ball on the way down, then repeat.

Woodchop slam

1. Stand with a wide stance.
2. Hold the slam ball and lift it up and away from your body to the left-hand side, rotating on the ball of your right foot.
3. Keeping your arms extended, rotate on the ball of your left foot and bring the slam ball down across your body and to your right hand. As you do this the heel of your right foot will return to the floor.
4. Reverse the movement, keeping your arms extended and rotating up and across your body to the left-hand side again.

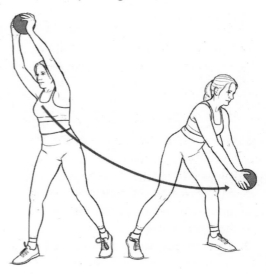

Rotation slam

1. Stand sideways to a wall, so that the left-hand side of your body is closest to it, arm's-length away, with feet hip distance apart and holding the slam ball, arms extended to the right-hand side.
2. Rotate your torso to the left, keeping your hips facing forwards, and explosively drive the slam ball into the wall.
3. Either catch the ball on the way down to repeat on the other side, or take a small step backwards and allow the ball to hit the ground before picking up and repeating.

The cooldown

Just as the warm-up plays an important role in preparing for exercise, the cooldown is essential to post-exercise recovery and restoring homeostasis. Homeostasis is a balanced state of all the body systems; several body systems are affected during exercise, including your breathing rate, heart rate, fluid balance, blood pressure, perspiration rate and body temperature. Muscles, tissues and joints are also affected. An adequate cooldown helps promote recovery to:

- Return heart rate and blood pressure to a pre-exercise state.
- Reduce muscle soreness.
- Prevent injury.
- Decrease the risk of blood pooling and fainting.
- Helps the mind and body to transition to a calm and relaxed state.

The type of cooldown you perform can depend on what the main exercise session included. For example, when I have been for a run my cooldown involves decreasing my running pace to a jog, then jogging slowly for the last 5 minutes of my run. I then follow this with stretches primarily for the lower body and legs, including developmental stretches for areas that I am restricted in or where I have muscle tightness.

When I work with a client who has completed a whole-body session, including cardiovascular exercises and strength and conditioning exercises, I take a different approach. This includes slowly lowering the pulse rate with some gently mobility moves for 3–5 minutes, followed by some assisted partner stretches and sometimes a guided meditation or relaxation exercise. Most cooldowns will take 8–10 minutes to complete, although they can be longer if several stretches focused on developing greater flexibility are required.

For most of the workouts included in this book I recommend you perform some slow body-weight cardiovascular moves over 2–3 minutes, such as walking on the spot and some gentle arm swings. This will start the process of returning your heart rate and blood pressure to your pre-exercise state, when coupled with post-exercise stretches.

Pulse-lowering exercises

These four exercises work well together as a pulse-lowering activity – three are from the whole-body warm-up section on page 148. Aim to slowly decrease the range of movement and the tempo with each exercise, so that you finish with some gentle heel-raise walking before moving on to the stretches. Complete each exercise for 45–60 seconds, 4–5 minutes in total.

Abdominals, back and shoulders

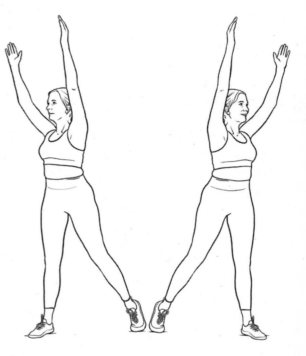

1. Widen your stance, then reach your hands upwards and across your body in a diagonal movement to your right, allowing your left heel to lift off the floor as you rotate through your torso. Feel the weight shift to your right leg.

2. Lengthen through your back at the same time so that your arms are outstretched from the top of your fingertips on your right, through to the toes on your left foot.

3. Now imagine you are tracing an upside-down rainbow as your hands lead the movement, arcing downwards and then upwards to your left-hand side.

4. As you do this your left heel returns to the floor so your left foot is balanced and flat, and your right heel lifts upwards as you pivot on the toes of your right foot.

5. Repeat this sweeping arc movement, slowly reducing the range of movement.

Standing reach to semi-squat with fingertip sweep

1. Stand with feet hip distance apart.
2. Raise your arms up overhead and rise onto your toes at the same time (if possible).
3. While performing a semi-squat movement – hinging at the hip and bending at the knees – flow your arms back downwards, keeping them straight, and try to sweep the floor with your fingertips.
4. Repeat, keeping the movement slow and gentle.

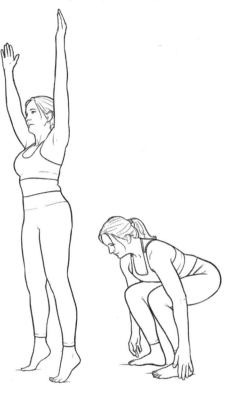

Walking on the spot

1. Lift one knee slightly to begin walking on the spot, but keep your toes in contact with the floor.
2. Lift the whole foot off the floor, then repeat, alternating with the other leg.
3. As you 'walk', allow your arms to swing naturally – opposite arm swings forwards to the raised knee.

Heel-raise walking

1. Stand with feet hip distance apart, with soft knees.
2. Bring one heel up slightly, keeping the forefoot and toes in contact with the floor, to begin heel-raise walking on the spot.
3. Allow your arms to swing naturally – opposite arm to opposite heel raise.

Why stretch?

The main benefit of stretching is to maintain or improve flexibility and the range of movement in a joint. Flexibility is a key component of fitness, and if it is restricted it will impact your ability to engage in other elements of fitness and daily life. For example, tight hamstrings can make it difficult to walk or even stand comfortably, while shoulder restrictions can make pressing and reaching movements overhead challenging.

Flexibility tends to decrease as we grow older, and there are several reasons for this, including lifestyle factors such as a general reduction in movement with age, lack of use and not stretching regularly. Structural changes in a joint, like osteoarthritis, can also limit range of movement.

As muscle ages, stretching, along with strength training, is crucial to maintain function and independence. At the most basic of needs this can make the difference in being able to reach and cut your own toenails, something many older adults struggle with.

Contained in this section, for the sake of simplicity and space, I am including a selection of key stretches for the whole body. This is not an exhaustive list as there are many different types of stretches, but I have selected those that are particularly beneficial as we grow older, with a special focus on areas of the body where we can start to develop restrictions.

Stretches can be performed while standing, seated on a chair or the floor, or lying down. The stretches described here are a mixture of all three. The order in which stretches are performed should flow naturally, which normally means the first one or two stretches are performed in a standing position, then you move onto the floor where you may do one or two seated stretches before performing lying stretches. With the lying stretches, avoid flipping from front to back and over again. Instead, group the stretches so that you perform all those lying face down, followed by those lying face up. Conclude your stretches by a seated stretch and a standing stretch.

When performing seated stretches on the floor I recommend you extend your legs, bending at the knees with feet flat on the floor in front on you. Sit on a Pilates block or cushion if preferred. Lying stretches should be performed on your exercise mat.

The stretches included here are static stretches to help either maintain or improve flexibility. The method for each is as follows:

1. Take a deep breath in to prepare for the stretch.
2. Initiate the stretch as you exhale.
3. Ease into the stretch until you feel mild tension.
4. Continue to breathe normally as you hold the stretch.
5. After about 10 seconds, take another deep breath in and try to ease a little further into the stretch.
6. Hold the stretch for 15–30 seconds minimum, up to a maximum of 60 seconds.

If you have completed a whole-body workout I recommend you follow the stretches in this order. These also work as part of a standalone stretch routine, but it's important not to stretch cold muscles, so always perform some gentle movements first, like the whole-body warm-up routine in this chapter.

If you struggle to reach a limb when instructed to hold onto one, use a towel or resistance band to assist. For example, on the lying hamstring stretch, if you can't reach your thigh to pull your leg into a stretch you could loop a towel behind your thigh and pull on that instead.

Stretches for the whole body

The following exercises include a range of stretches for the whole body. They can form part of your post-exercise recovery or work as standalone stretches, provided you have already completed a suitable warm-up.

Standing calf stretch

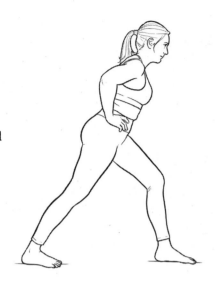

1. Stand with feet hip distance apart and take a big stride forward on your right foot.
2. Bend your right knee, keeping your left leg extended and straight – the position from your head to your left leg should make one straight line at around a 45-degree angle to the ground.
3. Change sides and repeat.

Standing doorway pec stretch

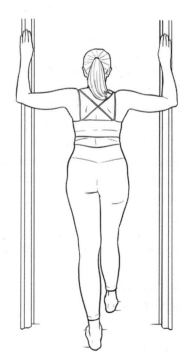

1. Stand in an open doorway and stagger your feet slightly for stability.
2. Lift your arms to shoulder height at the sides, with elbows at right angles and palms facing forwards.
3. Place and press your forearms on either side on the doorway frame, palms flat.
4. Step forwards into the doorway, easing yourself through as you feel the stretch in your chest.

Standing thoracic extension wall stretch

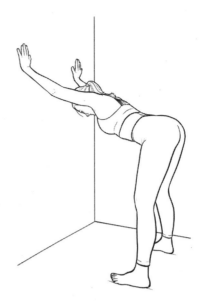

1. Stand facing a wall with outstretched arms at shoulder height.
2. Place your palms flat against the wall.
3. Keeping your hands flat, push the hips slightly backwards as you lower the chest downwards in a bowing movement.
4. Feel the shoulders stretch overhead as the middle and upper back extends.

Seated lateral neck stretch

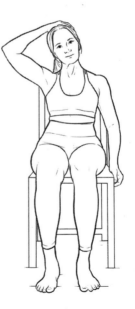

1. Sit with a neutral spine posture, hands rested at your sides.
2. Looking straight ahead, gently tilt your head sideways to the right. Decrease the distance between your right ear and right shoulder, keeping your shoulders straight and level throughout.
3. Assist the stretch by bringing your right arm over your head and cradling the left-hand side of your head with your right hand, applying gentle pressure as you do so.
4. Change sides and repeat.

Seated triceps stretch

1. Sit with a neutral spine posture.
2. Reach your right arm up and drop your right hand behind your head.
3. Keep the right elbow over your right shoulder.
4. With your left hand, apply gently pressure to your right upper arm and push into the stretch.
5. Alternatively, hold a towel in your right hand, drop the length of the towel behind your body, then hold and pull the other end of the towel with your left hand.

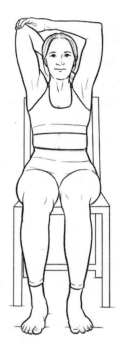

Child's pose

1. Kneel on all fours, then sit back on your heels, opening your thighs wider as you do so.
2. Stretch your arms and upper body out in front of you.
3. Sink your upper body between your open thighs, with palms flat on the floor.

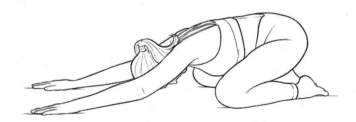

Thread the needle

1. Kneel on all fours.
2. Sit back on your heels, opening your thighs wider as you do so.
3. Stretch your arms and upper body out in front of you.

4. Exhale and bring your right arm underneath your left arm and shoulder with your palm facing upwards.

5. Rest the right side of your face on your exercise mat and look towards your outstretched right arm and hand.

6. Hold for 15–20 seconds before pushing back to all fours and changing sides.

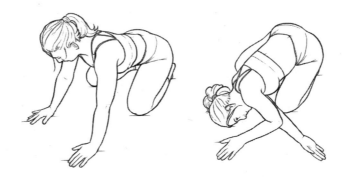

Lying quad and hip flexor stretch

1. Lie flat on the floor, face down.

2. Lift your left arm upwards, bending at the elbow, to rest on the floor.

3. Rest your forehead on your left arm.

4. Bending your right knee, hold your ankle with your right hand, and draw your heel in towards your buttocks.

5. Push your hips into the mat until you feel a stretch along the front of your thigh.

6. Repeat on the other side.

7. An alternative option is to perform this in a side-lying position, if preferred.

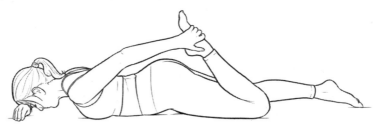

Lying thoracic rotation stretch

1. Lie on your back, arms outstretched with palms upwards, making a 'T' shape with your body.
2. Bend your right knee and cross your right foot over your left knee, resting it on the floor.
3. Rest your left hand on the side of your right knee and apply gentle pressure.
4. Turn your head to the right to look at your outstretched right arm.
5. Repeat on the other side.

Lying hamstring stretch

1. Lie on your back, bending both knees with the feet flat on the floor.
2. Lift and straighten your right leg upwards.
3. Hold on to the back of your right thigh with your hands and gently pull your leg towards your body, without bending the knee, until you feel a stretch down the back of your right leg. You can extend and straighten your left leg on the floor, if preferred, or loop a towel behind your thigh and pull the ends of the towel towards your body.
4. Repeat on the other side.

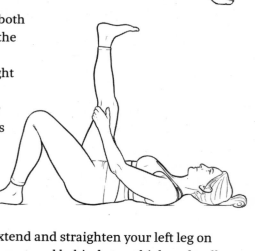

Seated inner groin stretch

1. Sit on the floor or elevated on a Pilates block or cushion, with a neutral spine posture.
2. Bring the soles of your feet together and, holding your ankles, pull them closer towards your groin.
3. Allow your knees to drop gently outwards and towards the ground as you feel the stretch in your inner groin.

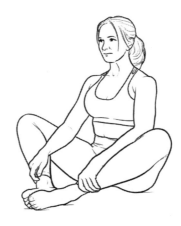

Seated glutes stretch with rotation

1. Sit with neutral spine posture, with your legs straight and extended to the front.
2. Bend your right knee, and with the foot flat on the floor draw it inwards in line with your left knee.
3. Lift your right foot and place it on the floor on the outer side on your left leg.
4. Rotate your torso round to the right and place your right hand on the floor behind your right-hand side.
5. Push the back of your left arm against the outside of your right bent leg.

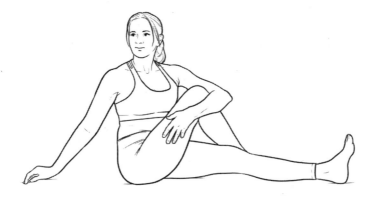

Seated shoulder stretch

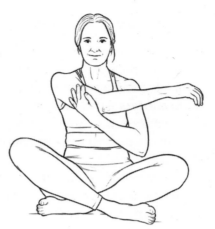

1. Sit with a neutral spine posture.
2. Bring your right arm across your body, and holding onto your right upper arm with your left hand, draw it closer to your body until you feel a stretch at the back of your shoulder.
3. Use the cradle of your left elbow to support your right arm.
4. Repeat on the other side.

Whole-body stretch

1. Lie on your back with your arms relaxed at your sides, palms up and legs extended and straight.
2. Inhale, and on the exhale focus on releasing any tension and imagine melting into the mat.
3. Relax your abdominal muscles.
4. Close your eyes (if this feels comfortable for you) and bring your focus to your breathing.

How to exercise for YOUR body – modifications and adaptations to popular exercises

There are numerous ways to make fitness accessible and inclusive to everyone; exercise can be modified and adapted to suit a wide range of abilities and needs. You only need to look to para-athletes for evidence that despite physical challenges many people not only engage in physical activity but compete in sporting endeavours at the highest level.

Throughout this book I have highlighted common ways in which you can modify and adapt exercises to suit you. Here are some alternative ways to modify exercises to make them easier to perform:

- Exercise in a seated position.
- Hold onto the back of a chair for additional support.
- Reduce the range of movement.
- Lower intensity.
- Exercise for a shorter period of time.
- Use lighter weights.
- Extend the warm-up.
- Take longer rest breaks between exercises.

Alternatively, here are a few ways by which you can modify exercises to make them harder:

- Exercise while standing.
- Use unilateral exercises.
- Focus on using a full range of movement.
- Increase the intensity.
- Extend duration.
- Use heavier weights.
- Perform multiple sets or more repetitions.
- Include minimal to no rest breaks.
- Wear a weighted vest.

It's not possible to include an exhaustive list of ways by which you can make the exercises in this book either easier or harder. Instead, remember these general principles and refer to the specific adaptations and modifications listed within each exercise segment for more details.

CHAPTER 10

WORK IT OUT

There are a variety of complete workouts included in this chapter, which are designed for all abilities from beginner through to intermediate and incorporate the exercises listed on pages 148 to 212.

These workouts and exercises will help you address the eleven components of fitness highlighted in Chapter 1, and are divided into those focused on strength, cardiovascular and core, and a circuit-based session which incorporates elements from all three. The strength workouts are further divided into whole body, upper body and lower body.

You'll also find agility training workouts here that incorporate fast footwork, as well as slam ball exercises for explosive power. There are also some suggestions for 'exercise snacks', too, when you need to slow things down and take a quick movement break.

Whole-body strength – beginner

Equipment: Dumbbells, exercise mat

Warm-up
Start by performing all the exercises in the whole-body warm-up on page 148.

Main session
Sets: 2   **Reps:** 8–12   **Rest:** 60 seconds
- Romanian deadlift (page 181)
- Goblet squats (page 183)
- Split squats (page 183)

- Chest press (page 193)
- Single arm row (page 185)
- Lateral raise (page 195)
- Biceps curls (page 194)
- Single arm triceps kickback (page 187)

Cooldown
- Standing calf stretch (page 206)
- Standing doorway pec stretch (page 206)
- Standing thoracic extension wall stretch (page 207)
- Seated triceps stretch (page 208)
- Child's pose (page 208)
- Lying quad and hip flexor stretch (page 209)
- Lying hamstring stretch (page 210)
- Seated inner groin stretch (page 211)
- Seated shoulder stretch (page 212)

Cardiovascular workout – beginner

Equipment: Exercise mat

Warm-up
Start by performing all the exercises in the whole-body warm-up on
page 148.

Main session
Perform the following exercises as a circuit:
Work for 30 seconds   Rest for 30 seconds
Circuits × 2 (rest 1–2 minutes after the first circuit) – remember to swap
sides, where relevant, on the second circuit.
- Heel-raise walking (page 203)
- Walking on the spot (page 203)
- Vertical rope pulls (page 159)
- Lateral lunge (page 184)
- Running arms (page 160)
- Half jacks (page 162)
- Rotation with jab (page 159)

- Walkouts (page 160)
- Side shuffles or steps (page 163)
- Mountain climbers (page 161)

Cooldown
- Complete all four of the pulse-lowering exercises (pages 201–203)
- Standing calf stretch (page 206)
- Standing doorway pec stretch (page 206)
- Standing thoracic extension wall stretch (page 207)
- Child's pose (page 208)
- Lying quad and hip flexor stretch (page 209)
- Lying hamstring stretch (page 210)
- Whole-body stretch (page 212)
- Seated glutes stretch with rotation (page 211)
- Seated inner groin stretch (page 211)

Core training – beginner

Equipment: Exercise mat

Warm-up
Start by performing the following four exercises to warm up and prepare for the main session:
- Walking on the spot for 2 minutes (cardiovascular exercise, page 157)
- Abdominals, back and shoulders (page 149)
- Hips, knees and ankles (page 149)
- Cat cow (page 153)

Main session
Sets: 2   **Reps:** 6–8   **Rest:** 60 seconds
- Abdominal hollowing (page 171)
- Ab curl (page 172)
- Back extension (page 172)
- Pelvic tilt (page 171)
- Low plank – kneeling (hold for 10–20 seconds) (page 175)
- Supine bridge (page 173)

Cooldown
- Cat cow (page 153)
- Child's pose (page 208)
- Seated glutes stretch with rotation (page 211)
- Whole-body stretch (page 212)

Circuit session – beginner

Equipment: Exercise mat

Warm-up
Start by performing all the exercises in the whole-body warm-up on page 148.

Main session
Perform the following exercises as a circuit:
Work for 30 seconds   Rest for 30 seconds
Circuits × 2 (rest for 1–2 minutes after the first circuit) – remember to swap sides, where relevant, on the second circuit.
- Walking on the spot (page 203)
- Squats (body weight) (page 168)
- Horizontal rope pulls (page 158)
- Reverse lunge (body weight) (page 169)
- Half jacks (page 162)
- Wall push or modified push-ups (page 167 or 168)
- Butt kicks (page 163)
- Floor dips (body weight) (page 170)
- Stepping skaters with knee touch (page 164)
- Supine heel tap or half get-up (page 173 or 178)

Cooldown
- Complete all four of the pulse-lowering exercises (page 201)
- Standing calf stretch (page 206)
- Standing doorway pec stretch (page 206)
- Standing thoracic extension wall stretch (page 207)
- Child's pose (page 208)

- Lying quad and hip flexor stretch (page 209)
- Lying hamstring stretch (page 210)
- Seated triceps stretch (page 208)
- Seated glutes stretch with rotation (page 211)
- Seated inner groin stretch (page 211)

Cardio and core combo – beginner

Equipment: Exercise mat

Warm-up
Start by performing all the exercises in the whole-body warm-up on
page 148.

Main cardiovascular session
Perform the following exercises as a circuit:
Work for 30 seconds   Rest for 30 seconds
Circuits × 2 (rest for 1–2 minutes after the first circuit) – remember to
swap sides, where relevant, on the second circuit.
- Walking on the spot (page 157)
- Vertical rope pulls (page 159)
- Lateral lunge (page 184)
- Walkouts (page 160)
- Rotation with jab (page 159)
- Half jacks (page 162)
- Side shuffles or steps (page 163)
- Mountain climbers (page 161)

Complete all four of the pulse-lowering exercises (page 201) before
moving on to the four core exercises.

Core exercises
Sets: 2   **Reps:** 6–8   **Rest:** 60 seconds
- Ab curl (page 172)
- Back extension (page 172)
- Supine bridge (page 173)
- Low plank – kneeling (hold for 10–20 seconds) (page 175)

Cooldown

- Child's pose (page 208)
- Lying quad and hip flexor stretch (page 209)
- Lying hamstring stretch (page 210)
- Whole-body stretch (page 212)
- Seated glutes stretch with rotation (page 211)
- Seated inner groin stretch (page 211)
- Standing doorway pec stretch (page 206)
- Standing thoracic extension wall stretch (page 207)
- Standing calf stretch (page 206)

Fast-feet agility workout – beginner

Equipment: Pilates block, exercise mat

Warm-up
Start by performing all the exercises in the whole-body warm-up on
page 148.

Main session
Perform the following exercises as a circuit:
Work for 30 seconds   Rest for 30 seconds
Circuits × 4 (rest for 1–2 minutes after the first circuit) – remember to
swap sides, where relevant, on each circuit.

- Half jacks (page 162)
- Fast feet (page 157)
- Standing knee drive with arms (page 164)
- Side toe taps (page 158)
- Mountain climbers (page 161)

Cooldown

- Complete all four of the pulse-lowering exercises (page 201)
- Standing calf stretch (page 206)
- Lying quad and hip flexor stretch (page 209)
- Lying hamstring stretch (page 210)

- Lying thoracic rotation stretch (page 210)
- Seated inner groin stretch (page 211)

Whole-body strength – intermediate

Equipment: Dumbbells, exercise mat

Warm-up
Start by performing all the exercises in the whole-body warm-up on page 148. Add the following exercises from the additional floor-based dynamic mobility exercises:
- All fours to downward dog (page 152)
- World's greatest stretch (page 154)

Main session
Sets: 3   **Reps:** 8–12   **Rest:** 60 seconds
- Deadlift (page 192)
- Clean and press (page 191)
- Goblet squats (page 183)
- Forward lunge (page 183)
- Chest press (page 193)
- Bent-over row (page 186)
- Triceps dips (page 188)
- Biceps curls (page 194)

Cooldown
- Standing calf stretch (page 206)
- Standing doorway pec stretch (page 206)
- Standing thoracic extension wall stretch (page 207)
- Seated triceps stretch (page 208)
- Child's pose (page 208)
- Lying quad and hip flexor stretch (page 209)
- Lying thoracic rotation stretch (page 210)
- Lying hamstring stretch (page 210)
- Seated inner groin stretch (page 211)
- Seated shoulder stretch (page 212)

Cardiovascular workout – intermediate

Equipment: Exercise mat

Warm-up
Start by performing all the exercises in the whole-body warm-up on page 148, followed by 1 minute of walkouts (page 160) and 2 minutes of walking on the spot (page 157), increasing to fast marching on the spot.

Main session
Perform the following exercises as a circuit:
Work for 40 seconds   Rest for 20 seconds
Circuits × 2 (rest for 1–2 minutes after the first circuit) – remember to swap sides, where relevant, on the second circuit.
- Vertical rope pulls (page 159)
- Lateral lunge with touchdown (page 158)
- Mock skipping (page 162)
- Half jacks (page 162)
- Rotation with jab and kick (page 160)
- Walkouts (page 160)
- Skaters with touchdown (page 163)
- Mountain climbers (page 161)
- Standing knee drive with arms (page 164)
- Plank jacks (page 166)

Cooldown
- Complete all four of the pulse-lowering exercises (page 201)
- Standing calf stretch (page 206)
- Standing doorway pec stretch (page 206)
- Standing thoracic extension wall stretch (page 207)
- Child's pose (page 208)
- Lying quad and hip flexor stretch (page 209)
- Lying hamstring stretch (page 210)
- Lying thoracic rotation stretch (page 210)

- Whole-body stretch (page 212)
- Seated inner groin stretch (page 211)

Core training – intermediate

Equipment: Exercise mat

Warm-up
Start by performing the following five exercises to warm up and prepare for the main session:
- Walking on the spot for 2 minutes (cardiovascular exercise, page 157)
- Abdominals, back and shoulders, and hips, knees and ankles (page 149)
- All fours to downward dog (page 152)
- Cat cow (page 153)
- World's greatest stretch (page 154)

Main session
Sets: 3   **Reps:** 6–8   **Rest:** 60 seconds
- Ab curl (page 172)
- Back extension (page 172)
- Supine bridge (page 173)
- Dead bug (page 174)
- Plank to knee tap (page 177)
- Half get-up (page 178)

Cooldown
- Hand behind head thoracic rotation (page 153)
- Child's pose (page 208)
- Lying thoracic rotation stretch (page 210)
- Whole-body stretch (page 212)

Circuit session – intermediate

Equipment: Dumbbells, exercise mat

Warm-up
Start by performing all the exercises in the whole-body warm-up
on page 148. Add in the following exercises from the additional
floor-based dynamic mobility exercises:
- All fours to downward dog (page 152)
- World's greatest stretch (page 153)

Main session
Perform the following exercises as a circuit:
Work for 40 seconds   Rest for 20 seconds
Circuits × 2 (rest for 1–2 minutes after the first circuit) – remember to
swap sides, where relevant, on the second circuit.
- Clean and press (page 191)
- Lateral lunge with touchdown (page 158)
- Goblet squats (page 183)
- Half jacks or jumping jacks (page 162)
- Forward lunge (page 183)
- Walk outs (page 160)
- Chest press or push ups (page 193 or 168)
- Crab toe reach (page 179)
- Triceps kickbacks (page 187)
- Get-up (page 178)

Cooldown
- Complete all four of the pulse-lowering exercises (page 201)
- Standing calf stretch (page 206)
- Standing doorway pec stretch (page 206)
- Standing thoracic extension wall stretch (page 207)
- Child's pose (page 208)
- Lying quad and hip flexor stretch (page 209)
- Lying hamstring stretch (page 210)
- Lying thoracic rotation stretch (page 210)

- Seated triceps stretch (page 208)
- Seated inner groin stretch (page 211)

Cardio and core combo – intermediate

Equipment: Exercise mat

Warm-up
Start by performing all the exercises in the whole-body warm up on page 148.

Main cardiovascular session
Perform the following exercises as a circuit:
Work for 40 seconds   Rest for 20 seconds
Circuits × 2 (rest for 1–2 minutes after the first circuit) – remember to swap sides, where relevant, on the second circuit.
- Marching or running on the spot (page 157)
- Squat drives or squat jumps (page 165)
- Lateral lunge with touchdown (page 158)
- Walkouts (page 160)
- Rotation with jab and kick (page 160)
- Half jacks (page 162)
- Skaters with touchdown (page 163)
- Mountain climbers (page 161)

Complete all four of the pulse-lowering exercises (page 201) before moving onto the four core exercises.

Core exercises
Sets: 2   **Work:** 40 seconds   **Rest:** 20 seconds
- Alternate supine heel taps (page 174)
- Crab toe reach (page 179)
- Plank to foot tap (page 177)
- Get-up (page 178)

Cooldown
- Child's pose (page 208)
- Lying quad and hip flexor stretch (page 209)
- Lying hamstring stretch (page 210)
- Whole-body stretch (page 212)
- Lying thoracic rotation stretch (page 210)
- Seated inner groin stretch (page 211)
- Standing doorway pec stretch (page 206)
- Standing thoracic extension wall stretch (page 207)
- Standing calf stretch (page 206)

Fast-feet agility workout – intermediate

Equipment: Pilates block, exercise mat

Warm up
Start by performing all the exercises in the whole-body warm-up on
  page 148.

Main session
Perform the following exercises as a circuit:
Work for 40 seconds   Rest for 20 seconds
Circuits × 2 (rest for 1–2 minutes after the first circuit) – remember to
swap sides, where relevant, on the second circuit.
- Butt kicks (page 163)
- Standing knee drive with arms (page 164)
- Side toe taps (page 158)
- Fast feet (page 157)
- Toe taps to Pilates block (page 158)
- Mock skipping (page 162)
- Half jacks or jumping jacks (page 162)
- Skaters with touchdown (page 163)
- Mountain climbers (page 161)
- Plank jacks (page 166)

Cooldown

- Complete all four of the pulse-lowering exercises (page 201)
- Standing calf stretch (page 206)
- Lying quad and hip flexor stretch (page 209)
- Lying hamstring stretch (page 210)
- Lying thoracic rotation stretch (page 210)
- Seated inner groin stretch (page 211)

Slam ball workout – intermediate

Equipment: Slam ball, exercise mat

Warm-up
Start by performing all the exercises in the whole-body warm-up on
page 148.

Main session
Perform the following exercises as a circuit:
Work for 40 seconds   Rest for 20 seconds
Circuits × 4 (rest for 1–2 minutes after the first circuit) – remember to
swap sides, where relevant, on the second circuit.

- Overhead slam (page 198)
- Rotation slam (page 200)
- Squat throw (page 199)
- Rainbow slam (page 198)
- Squat to wall ball slam (page 199)
- Woodchop slam (page 200)

Cooldown

- Complete all four of the pulse-lowering exercises on
  pages 201–203
- Cat cow (page 153)
- Hand behind head thoracic rotation (page 153)
- Child's pose (page 208)
- Lying quad and hip flexor stretch (page 209)
- Lying hamstring stretch (page 210)

- Lying thoracic rotation stretch (page 210)
- Seated inner groin stretch (page 211)
- Standing thoracic extension wall stretch (page 207)
- Standing doorway pec stretch (page 206)
- Whole-body stretch (page 212)
- Standing calf stretch (page 206)
- Seated triceps stretch (page 208)
- Seated glutes stretch with rotation (page 212)
- Seated shoulder stretch (page 212)
- Seated lateral neck stretch (page 207)

Additional workouts

These additional workouts do not feature in the beginner and intermediate weekly plans in the next chapter. However, they are included here as options for when you are travelling, nursing a lower- or upper body injury, or need something short and sweet on days when you can't face a full session or only have 15 minutes to spare.

Resistance bands are a user-friendly option for beginners, as they are easier to hold if you have grip issues, and ideal for travelling as they are light and portable.

Whole-body strength with resistance bands – beginner

Equipment: Resistance bands, exercise mat

Warm-up
Start by performing all the exercises in the whole-body warm-up on page 148.

Main session
Sets: 2   **Reps:** 8–12   **Rest:** 60 seconds
- Deadlift (page 192)
- Squats (page 193)

- Seated row (page 194)
- Chest press (page 193)
- Split squats (page 169)
- Pulldown (page 196)
- Lateral raise (page 195)
- Biceps curls (page 194)
- Single arm triceps extension (page 195)

Splitting your training into upper body strength days and lower body strength days is a technique used by bodybuilders. However, it is also a helpful option if you have a niggle or an injury. The following upper body or lower body strength sessions enable you to carry on strength training even when you may need to rest a particular area of the body.

Upper body strength – beginner

Equipment: Dumbbells, exercise mat

Warm-up
Start by performing the following warm-up exercises from the whole-body warm-up:
- Neck and head (page 148)
- Shoulders (page 148)
- Chest and upper back (page 149)
- Abdominals, back and shoulders (page 149)

Main session
Sets: 2   **Reps:** 8–12   **Rest:** 60 seconds
- Wall push or countertop push up (page 167)
- Single arm row (page 185)
- Shoulder press (page 189)
- Reverse fly (page 190)
- Biceps curls (page 194)
- Single arm triceps kickback (page 187)

Cooldown
- Standing doorway pec stretch (page 206)
- Standing thoracic extension wall stretch (page 207)
- Seated triceps stretch (page 208)
- Child's pose (page 208)
- Seated shoulder stretch (page 212)
- Seated lateral neck stretch (page 207)

Lower body strength – beginner

Equipment: Dumbbells, exercise mat

Warm-up
Start by performing the following warm-up exercises from the whole-body warm-up:
- Ankles (page 151)
- Hips (page 150)
- Legs (back of thighs) (page 150)
- Legs (front of thighs) and knees (page 150)
- Legs, back, abdominals and shoulders (page 150)

Main session
Sets: 2 **Reps:** 8–12 **Rest:** 60 seconds
- Squats (body weight) (page 168)
- Romanian deadlift (page 181)
- Split squats (page 169)
- Lateral lunge (page 184)
- Pelvic tilt (page 171)
- Supine bridge (page 173)

Cooldown
- Standing calf stretch (page 206)
- Lying quad and hip flexor stretch (page 209)
- Lying hamstring stretch (page 210)
- Lying thoracic rotation stretch (page 210)
- Seated inner groin stretch (page 211)

Upper body strength – intermediate

Equipment: Dumbbells, exercise mat

Warm-up
Start by performing the following warm-up exercises from the whole-body warm-up:
- Neck and head (page 148)
- Shoulders (page 148)
- Chest and upper back (page 149)
- Cat cow (page 153)
- All fours to downward dog (page 152)
- World's greatest stretch (page 154)

Main session
Sets: 3   **Reps:** 8–12   **Rest:** 60 seconds
- Modified push ups or push ups (page 168)
- Bent-over row (page 186)
- Triceps dips (page 188)
- Reverse fly (page 190)
- Shoulder press (page 189)
- Biceps curls (page 194)

Cooldown
- Standing doorway pec stretch (page 206)
- Standing thoracic extension wall stretch (page 207)
- Seated triceps stretch (page 208)
- Child's pose (page 208)
- Lying thoracic rotation stretch (page 210)
- Seated shoulder stretch (page 212)
- Seated lateral neck stretch (page 207)

Lower body strength – intermediate

Equipment: Dumbbells, exercise mat

Warm-up
Start by performing the following warm-up exercises from the whole-body warm-up:
- Ankles (page 151)
- Hips (page 150)
- Hips, back, legs and bottom (page 150)
- Legs, back, abdominals and shoulders (page 150)
- Half-kneeling lunge to hamstring stretch (page 155)
- Adductor rock back (page 155)

Main session
Sets: 3   **Reps:** 8–12   **Rest:** 60 seconds
- Deadlift (page 192)
- Squats (page 168)
- Forward lunge (page 183)
- Lateral lunge (page 184)
- Single leg deadlift (page 182)
- Supine bridge (page 173)

Cooldown
- Standing calf stretch (page 206)
- Lying quad and hip flexor stretch (page 209)
- Lying hamstring stretch (page 210)
- Lying thoracic rotation stretch (page 210)
- Seated glutes stretch with rotation (page 211)
- Seated inner groin stretch (page 211)

Exercise snacks

There are many times when you might recognise that you need to move but you don't have time for a full workout. These exercise snacks are an ideal way to get some movement into your day, to break up extended sedentary periods, and to feel more energised. Take them at a gentle, easy pace, as they are not intended to take the place of a full workout but simply offer an opportunity to move. Each will take under 10 minutes to complete.

Exercise snack 1

Complete 40 seconds of each exercise, resting between each movement as needed.

From the whole-body warm-up:
- Abdominals, back and shoulders (page 149)
- Legs, back, abdominals and shoulders (page 150)
- Hips (page 150)

From the cardiovascular exercises:
- Walking on the spot (page 157)
- Half jacks (page 162)

From the body-weight strength exercises:
- Squats (page 168)
- Reverse lunge (page 169)

From the pulse-lowering exercises:
- Standing reach to semi-squat with fingertip sweep (page 203)

Exercise snack 2

Complete 40 seconds of each exercise, resting between each movement as needed.

From the whole body warm-up:
- Floor angel (page 154)
- Cat cow (page 153)
- All fours to downward dog (page 152)

From the cardiovascular exercises:
- Walkouts (page 160)

From the core body-weight exercises:
- Bird dog (page 175)
- Plank to knee tap (page 177)

From the stretches for the whole body (hold for 30 seconds each):
- Child's pose (page 208)
- Whole body stretch (page 212)

Exercise snack 3

Complete 40 seconds of each exercise, resting between each movement as needed.

From the whole-body warm-up:
- Neck and head (page 148)
- Shoulders (page 148)
- Chest and back (page 149)
- Legs (back of thighs) (page 150)
- Legs (inner and outer thigh) (page 151)

From the cardiovascular exercises:
- Side toe taps (page 158)

From the pulse-lowering exercises:
- Abdominals, back and shoulders (page 202)

CHAPTER 11

YOUR WEEKLY PLAN

Details of all the workouts contained in the beginner and intermediate programmes can be found in Chapter 9. Each workout has been designed to take you less than 30 minutes, including the warm-up and cooldown. If you want to combine workouts (other than the combinations you'll find in Chapter 10), such as whole-body strength and core training, you are free to do so. This will increase the total length of session time, but it could give you an additional rest day. If you want to do this, I recommend you stick with the programme as it is for weeks 1–4, as these already have three rest days, and you do not drop down to less than three sessions each week, aiming to remain at four or five sessions per week whenever possible.

Beginner programme

If you are completely new to exercise or are returning to exercise after a long break, I recommend you start here. The beginner programme takes place over 12 weeks and has two phases. If you recall the principle of progressive overload from Chapter 8, your body will adapt and make physiological changes in strength and cardiovascular conditioning over a 6 to 8-week period. So, each phase lasts six weeks. However, if you get to week 6 and feel like you need to spend further time at this level, please repeat week 6 until you feel ready to move on. Likewise, if you need to take time off due to illness, work commitments or a holiday, then stay at your previous level for another week or two until you feel ready to progress. If you miss a workout, pick up the planned session you missed on your next workout day. Use the weekly plans just as a guide – they are not set in stone!

Beginner programme: Phase 1

This programme aims to ease you into regular exercise over a six-week period. In the first two weeks you'll complete three workouts, spaced throughout the week with rest days in between, giving you plenty of time to recover. You don't have to do the workouts on the days of the week specified; for example, day one of week 1 could start on a Tuesday or any other day of the week. Aim to keep the basic structure the same, though, with a workout day followed by a rest day, rather than doing the workouts three days in a row followed by a four-day gap.

If you are an absolute beginner or are returning to exercise after a long break, I would urge you to resist doing more workouts than those specified for the first two weeks. You may start off with great enthusiasm and want to do more workouts, but the best way to embed a regular exercise habit is to build it up gradually. In my experience, one of the biggest mistakes people make when they are new to exercise is doing too much too soon. Feeling highly motivated is common, but motivation can quickly wane, and I don't want you to rely on it. Instead, I want you to seamlessly integrate regular exercise into your routine and stick with it for the rest of your life. Starting gradually like this also reduces the risk of injury whilst you get familiar with the workouts.

There's no need to avoid all activity on rest days, though, as these days can be used for something known as active recovery. Active recovery involves low-intensity physical activity, such as walking, cycling, swimming, gardening or stretching – like the whole-body stretch routine on page 148.

On weeks 3 and 4 you'll drop one of the rest days and gain an additional beginner whole-body strength session. Performing these two whole-body strength sessions a week will bring you in line with the CMO's recommendations outlined in Chapter 8.

You'll drop down to two rest days on weeks 5 and 6 and gain an additional beginner cardiovascular workout. If you are including active recovery into your rest days, such as 2 × 20 minutes of brisk walking, or 40 minutes of gardening and 20 minutes of cycling, you'll now be achieving the CMO's recommendations for cardiovascular activity.

Week 1

Monday	Tuesday	Wednesday	Thursday	Friday	Saturday	Sunday
Beginner whole-body strength	Rest day	Beginner cardiovascular workout	Rest day	Beginner core training	Rest day or Whole-body stretch	Rest day

Week 2

Monday	Tuesday	Wednesday	Thursday	Friday	Saturday	Sunday
Beginner whole-body strength	Rest day	Beginner cardiovascular workout	Rest day	Beginner core training	Rest day or whole-body stretch	Rest day

Week 3

Monday	Tuesday	Wednesday	Thursday	Friday	Saturday	Sunday
Beginner whole-body strength	Beginner cardiovascular workout	Rest day	Beginner whole-body strength	Beginner core training	Rest day or whole-body stretch	Rest day

Week 4						
Monday	**Tuesday**	**Wednesday**	**Thursday**	**Friday**	**Saturday**	**Sunday**
Beginner whole-body strength	Beginner cardiovascular workout	Rest day	Beginner whole-body strength	Beginner core training	Rest day or whole-body stretch	Rest day

Week 5						
Monday	**Tuesday**	**Wednesday**	**Thursday**	**Friday**	**Saturday**	**Sunday**
Beginner whole-body strength	Beginner cardiovascular workout	Rest day or whole-body stretch	Beginner whole-body strength	Beginner cardiovascular workout	Beginner core training	Rest day

Week 6						
Monday	**Tuesday**	**Wednesday**	**Thursday**	**Friday**	**Saturday**	**Sunday**
Beginner whole-body strength	Beginner cardiovascular workout	Rest day or whole-body stretch	Beginner whole-body strength	Beginner cardiovascular workout	Beginner core training	Rest day

Beginner programme: Phase 2

This phase builds on the fitness foundation acquired over the first six weeks. In weeks 7 and 8 the twice-weekly beginner cardiovascular workout has been replaced with a new workout, the beginner cardio and core combo. Don't worry, it won't take you twice as long to complete, as it doesn't combine all the exercises from the beginner cardiovascular workout and core training, but a collection of them. The rest days remain at two, but instead of a dedicated core workout day, you now have a whole-body stretch session (alongside the optional whole-body stretch day on your first rest day of the week).

In weeks 9 and 10 the whole-body stretch day is replaced with another new workout, the beginner circuit session, and in weeks 11 and 12 this is replaced with your final new workout in this block, the fast-feet agility workout.

As in phase 1, use this programme as a guide. If you need to stay longer on a particular week, repeat the next week until you feel ready to progress.

Week 7						
Monday	**Tuesday**	**Wednesday**	**Thursday**	**Friday**	**Saturday**	**Sunday**
Beginner whole-body strength	Beginner cardio and core combo	Rest day or whole-body stretch	Beginner whole-body strength	Beginner cardio and core combo	Whole-body stretch	Rest day

Week 8						
Monday	**Tuesday**	**Wednesday**	**Thursday**	**Friday**	**Saturday**	**Sunday**
Beginner whole-body strength	Beginner cardio and core combo	Rest day or whole-body stretch	Beginner whole-body strength	Beginner cardio and core combo	Whole-body stretch	Rest day

Week 9						
Monday	**Tuesday**	**Wednesday**	**Thursday**	**Friday**	**Saturday**	**Sunday**
Beginner whole-body strength	Beginner cardio and core combo	Rest day or whole-body stretch	Beginner whole-body strength	Beginner cardio and core combo	Beginner circuit session	Rest day

Week 10

Monday	Tuesday	Wednesday	Thursday	Friday	Saturday	Sunday
Beginner whole-body strength	Beginner cardio and core combo	Rest day or whole-body stretch	Beginner whole-body strength	Beginner cardio and core combo	Beginner circuit session	Rest day

Week 11

Monday	Tuesday	Wednesday	Thursday	Friday	Saturday	Sunday
Beginner whole-body strength	Beginner cardio and core combo	Rest day or whole-body stretch	Beginner whole-body strength	Beginner cardio and core combo	Beginner fast-feet agility workout	Rest day

Week 12

Monday	Tuesday	Wednesday	Thursday	Friday	Saturday	Sunday
Beginner whole-body strength	Beginner cardio and core combo	Rest day or whole-body stretch	Beginner whole-body strength	Beginner cardio and core combo	Beginner fast-feet agility workout	Rest day

Congratulations, you have now completed the 12-week beginner programme. During these 12 weeks you have engaged in a range of exercises and workouts to support your cardiovascular health, strength and functional ability, mobility, flexibility and agility.

Progress isn't always linear. There will be times when you feel like you are making progress every single week, other times you might notice a plateau for a few weeks, and there will also be times when you regress a little – especially if you catch a virus or other illness that lasts more than a few days. Remember, you are in this for the long run, this isn't about quick fixes but establishing a lifelong habit of regular exercise as an active ager.

At this point review your progress to date, take stock and decide if you are ready to tackle the intermediate programme or whether you need more time to work through the beginner workouts. The choice is yours.

Intermediate programme

This intermediate programme introduces you to some new exercises that progress and build on the exercises you mastered in the beginner programme.

Intermediate programme: Phase 1

In the first two weeks you'll start off with three rest days again. This will help you adjust to the new increased workload of both the intermediate whole-body strength and cardiovascular workouts and learn some of the new exercises. Which means you have a total of four training sessions in weeks one and two, with an optional whole-body stretch session on two out of your three rest days. As with the beginner programme, I'd encourage you to use your rest days for active recovery and low-intensity physical activity, such as walking.

After these initial two weeks an additional session is introduced in weeks three and four, bringing your total weekly training sessions back to four, with two rest days.

In week 3 we reintroduce a fast-feet agility workout at an intermediate level. Look at your programme as a two-week block now for weeks 3 and 4, and weeks 5 and 6. This means that over two weeks you will complete three cardiovascular workouts, four strength workouts, four optional whole-body stretch sessions, one fast-feet agility workout, one core training and one circuit session – all at intermediate level. Although this might look like a decrease in cardiovascular sessions, both the circuit and fast-feet agility sessions have a cardiovascular training effect.

As with the beginner programme, phase 1 of the intermediate programme is a guide. If you don't feel ready to move on to the next week, simply repeat the week you are comfortable with. You also have the option to mix and match workouts between the beginner and intermediate programmes. For example, you could continue to do the beginner cardiovascular workouts but move on to the intermediate whole-body strength workout in week 1 if you feel more confident with your progress in strength training.

	Monday	Tuesday	Wednesday	Thursday	Friday	Saturday	Sunday
Week 1	Intermediate whole-body strength	Intermediate cardiovascular workout	Rest day or whole-body stretch	Intermediate whole-body strength	Intermediate cardiovascular workout	Rest day or whole-body stretch	Rest day
Week 2	Intermediate whole-body strength	Intermediate cardiovascular workout	Rest day or whole-body stretch	Intermediate whole-body strength	Intermediate cardiovascular workout	Rest day or whole-body stretch	Rest day
Week 3	Intermediate whole-body strength	Intermediate fast-feet agility workout	Rest day or whole-body stretch	Intermediate whole-body strength	Intermediate cardiovascular workout	Intermediate core training	Rest day

Week 4

Monday	Tuesday	Wednesday	Thursday	Friday	Saturday	Sunday
Intermediate whole-body strength	Intermediate cardiovascular workout	Rest day or whole-body stretch	Intermediate whole-body strength	Intermediate cardiovascular workout	Intermediate circuit session	Rest day

Week 5

Monday	Tuesday	Wednesday	Thursday	Friday	Saturday	Sunday
Intermediate whole-body strength	Intermediate fast-feet agility workout	Rest day or whole-body stretch	Intermediate whole-body strength	Intermediate cardiovascular workout	Intermediate core training	Rest day

Week 6

Monday	Tuesday	Wednesday	Thursday	Friday	Saturday	Sunday
Intermediate whole-body strength	Intermediate cardiovascular workout	Rest day or whole-body stretch	Intermediate whole-body strength	Intermediate cardiovascular workout	Intermediate circuit session	Rest day

Intermediate programme: Phase 2

The first two weeks of phase 2 repeats weeks 5 and 6 of phase 1. You will then work in two-week blocks for weeks nine and 10, and 11 and 12. In week 9 you have the option of introducing a slam ball workout – depending on whether you have a slam ball – or sticking with the fast-feet agility workout. In week 10 you'll discover a new combined cardiovascular and core workout, and another option to choose a circuit session or a slam ball workout. Weeks 11 and 12 are repeats of weeks 9 and 10.

Week 7

Monday	Tuesday	Wednesday	Thursday	Friday	Saturday	Sunday
Intermediate whole-body strength	Intermediate fast-feet agility workout	Rest day or whole-body stretch	Intermediate whole-body strength	Intermediate cardiovascular workout	Intermediate core training	Rest day

Week 8

Monday	Tuesday	Wednesday	Thursday	Friday	Saturday	Sunday
Intermediate whole-body strength	Intermediate cardiovascular workout	Rest day or whole-body stretch	Intermediate whole-body strength	Intermediate cardiovascular workout	Intermediate circuit session	Rest day

Week 9

Monday	Tuesday	Wednesday	Thursday	Friday	Saturday	Sunday
Intermediate whole-body strength	Intermediate fast-feet agility workout Or Slam ball workout	Rest day or whole-body stretch	Intermediate whole-body strength	Intermediate cardiovascular workout	Intermediate core training	Rest day

Week 10						
Monday	**Tuesday**	**Wednesday**	**Thursday**	**Friday**	**Saturday**	**Sunday**
Intermediate whole-body strength	Intermediate cardiovascular and core workout	Rest day or whole-body stretch	Intermediate whole-body strength	Intermediate cardiovascular workout	Intermediate circuit session Or Slam ball workout	Rest day

Week 11						
Monday	**Tuesday**	**Wednesday**	**Thursday**	**Friday**	**Saturday**	**Sunday**
Intermediate whole-body strength	Intermediate fast-feet agility workout Or Slam ball workout	Rest day or whole-body stretch	Intermediate whole-body strength	Intermediate cardiovascular workout	Intermediate core training	Rest day

Week 12						
Monday	**Tuesday**	**Wednesday**	**Thursday**	**Friday**	**Saturday**	**Sunday**
Intermediate whole-body strength	Intermediate cardiovascular and core workout	Rest day or whole-body stretch	Intermediate whole-body strength	Intermediate cardiovascular workout	Intermediate circuit session Or Slam ball workout	Rest day

Congratulations, you have now completed the 12-week intermediate programme. During these 12 weeks you have added to the range of strength-training exercises in your repertoire. You have engaged in exercises in multiple planes of movement. You've worked on your agility, balance, explosive power and functional movement patterns that support active ageing.

It's time to reflect on your journey so far and think about your next steps. If the weights you've been working with have become easier, you may want to invest in heavier ones. If you've found some of the exercises or workouts more challenging than others, you could try focusing on those over the next few weeks. There are enough exercises and workouts in this book to support your onward journey, and countless ways in which you could combine the exercises in this book to vary your training for the rest of your life – you just need to keep going!

CHAPTER 12

REHAB EXERCISES

By the time we reach our forties and fifties many of us will have experienced a joint injury or other musculoskeletal issue. An injury or a joint problem can be very frustrating and challenging, and in some cases, where activity is reduced in response to the issue, further health issues develop due to an increase in sedentary behaviour, activity becomes harder to engage in leading to further withdrawal, and so the downward health spiral continues.

A downward health spiral could easily have been my story. I have felt frustrated at times with the physical challenges to my health. I have had to come to terms with some of these challenges and accept the loss of what my body used to be able to do, without protesting too much! Despite some of the physical challenges I have faced over the past 20 years, I know how important it is to work around issues and how quickly our health trajectory can change if we fail to act. I've learnt first-hand the importance of prehab exercises (to prevent injury) and rehab exercises (to recover post injury or after a surgical procedure).

I'm always astounded at how many people muddle along with an injury or a niggle for months, and even years, before seeking a medical opinion. 'Assess don't guess' is a popular phrase used in the fitness industry; it emphasises the role of fitness tests and assessments in determining safe and effective exercise prescription. The human body is amazing at healing, given time, but 'assess don't guess' is relevant to remember if something isn't resolving. A medical assessment and diagnosis may be required and can help you make informed choices about your health.

This is especially relevant when you are engaged in physical activity, so that you can avoid movements or specific exercises that may exacerbate an issue. For example, with some knee issues a seated leg extension exercise may be contraindicated. An assessment and diagnosis can also help identify specific exercises to help improve function or manage pain – such as strengthening the quad muscles with knee osteoarthritis.

Assuming you've had an assessment and been given the green light to exercise (despite your condition causing some pain or discomfort), let's look at how to approach this from an active-ageing perspective.

How to approach pain

Pain is a warning sign, but knowing how to read pain signals and respond accordingly is important. It is understandable to want to avoid discomfort and reduce activity, with some conditions. You may fear making a condition worse or injuring yourself, but spending more time being sedentary, and reducing activity levels, can be counterproductive, leading to more health issues and further pain and discomfort. If you experience some degree of low-level background pain in your day-to-day life this is unlikely to vanish during exercise. Monitoring any changes to pain and discomfort, during and after exercise, is an important strategy in the management of many conditions.

The Visual Analog Scale (VAS) is a helpful tool to refer to when assessing pain and discomfort. The scale ranges from 0 to 10, where 0 = no pain and 10 = the worst pain possible. Using this scale as a method of self-evaluation during and after exercise will help boost your confidence in being physically active and working around any issue you encounter.

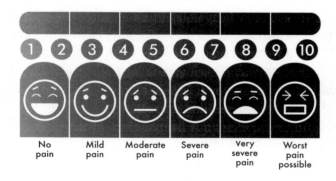

| No pain | Mild pain | Moderate pain | Severe pain | Very severe pain | Worst pain possible |

Here are four rules to follow during and after exercise if you live with some low level of background pain in your day-to-day life.

Rule 1

Whilst engaging in physical activity and exercise any pain or discomfort should be less than 4 on the VAS. Staying beneath 4 should help avoid making a problem worse.

Stop and do not continue if you experience pain above 4 on the VAS.

Rule 2

During exercise any pain should remain within your normal levels or decrease. Stop and do not continue if pain increases on the VAS during exercise.

Rule 3

Any pain or discomfort felt during exercise should either completely go or return to your usual baseline level as soon as you stop. Do not continue if pain experienced during exercise doesn't return to pre-exercise levels on the VAS.

Rule 4

Monitor any pain and discomfort in the first 24–48 hours after exercise. Any increase in pain needs to be reviewed. If exercise is new to you, or you are performing a new type of exercise, you may experience muscular soreness. This is known as delayed onset muscle soreness – DOMS – which normally peaks after 24–48 hours before subsiding and eventually going. An increase in pain in a joint may indicate that the intensity was too challenging for you, and reducing intensity may be helpful. Stop and modify exercise intensity if joint pain is increased in the 24–48 hours following exercise on the VAS.

Musculoskeletal signs and symptoms

Musculoskeletal pain is common during the menopause transition. Largely influenced by oestrogen flux, symptoms can include joint pain and stiffness known as arthralgia.[1]

In recent years a new term, the musculoskeletal syndrome of menopause, has been proposed by orthopaedic surgeon Dr Vonda Wright in a review paper of the same name published in March 2024.[2] The review calls for wider recognition of this term, and the collective musculoskeletal signs and symptoms women can experience during the menopause transition including musculoskeletal pain, arthralgia, reduction in lean muscle, loss of bone density, adhesive capsulitis and progression of osteoarthritis.

At the moment there is insufficient research to recommend strategies to prevent these musculoskeletal signs and symptoms. Many menopause experts believe a holistic approach to menopause is important in addressing these musculoskeletal signs and symptoms, and that Hormone Replacement Treatment (HRT) may also play a role. However, at present there is insufficient data and therefore no recommendation to start systemic HRT specifically for the prevention or treatment of osteoarthritis or adhesive capsulitis.

Whether you have a temporary or permanent joint issue there's nearly always a way to exercise and work around it. This is why I have included seated upper body strength workouts in Chapter 8, so you have options and can avoid a spiral of physical decline should you experience a challenge like this. Likewise, there are two lower body workouts, for times when you need to rest the upper body.

It would be impossible to cover an extensive range of musculoskeletal issues you might encounter in this chapter. Instead, let's look at three very common problems, which affect more women than men, especially those over the age of 40 – osteoarthritis, frozen shoulder and heel pain. I've worked with numerous clients who have experienced these conditions, and I have had first-hand experience of all three as well.

Plantar fasciopathy (heel pain)

I first developed heel pain in my late forties when I was training for the London Marathon. Plantar fasciopathy (PF) is a common cause of foot pain, which affects more women than men, and mostly occurs between the ages of 40 and 60. The lifetime prevalence of PF is estimated to be as high as 10 per cent, which means many of us may suffer this frustrating and debilitating condition. The plantar fascia is a band of tissue that stretches underneath the foot from the heel to the toes. In PF a dull ache or sharp pain is felt in the heel and underside of the foot. It can last just a few weeks, or in some cases many years.[3]

Plantar fasciopathy is associated with tightness in the calf muscle. This is due to tension exerted by the calf muscle, known as the gastrocnemius, as it pulls on the heel bone. This in turn pulls on the plantar fascia. Stretching and strengthening the calves is generally recognised as an important strategy in tackling heel pain.

Whether you currently have heel pain or you want to reduce your risk of developing foot and heel problems, the following exercises can be helpful in both working on your ankle flexibility and strength.

Warm up the ankles and calf muscles before performing stretches by using the ankle mobility exercise in the whole-body warm-up on page 148, for 60 seconds.

Ankles

1. Keeping your toes on the floor, lift one heel off the floor before gently lowering and lifting your other heel.
2. Pedal your heels alternately, lifting and lowering.
3. Follow this with the standing calf stretch in Chapter 8. Hold the stretch for 30 seconds, rest, change sides, then repeat for three rounds in total.

Standing calf stretch

1. Stand with feet hip distance apart and take a big stride forward on your right foot.

2. Bend your right knee, keeping your left leg extended and straight – your head to your left leg should make one straight line at around a 45-degree angle to the ground.
3. Change sides and repeat.

Alternatively, perform a seated calf stretch by looping a towel under your shoe, straightening your leg, and pulling the ball of your foot towards you.

Heel raises are often recommended to both strengthen ankle flexion and foot strength.[4]

Level 1: Isometric heel raises

Sets: 3   **Hold:** 30–60 seconds
1. Stand with feet hip distance apart.
2. Lift your heels upwards by pushing through the balls of your feet.
3. Hold for 30–60 seconds before gently lowering yourself down.

Level 2: Heel raises from a flat surface

Sets: 3   **Reps:** 8–12
1. Stand with feet hip distance apart.
2. Lift your heels upwards by pushing through the balls of your feet, pause, then hold for 2 seconds before lowering yourself down.
3. Repeat.

Level 3: Unilateral heel raises from an elevated surface

Sets: 3   **Reps:** 8–12
1. Use a step or put a couple of thick sturdy books on the floor.
2. Roll up a small towel and put it on the step or books.
3. Hold onto the back of a chair or wall for support.
4. Stand on the step or books with just the ball of your foot, and the rolled-up towel under your toes.

5. Bend the knee on your non-working leg.
6. Pushing through the ball of your working leg, rise up onto your toes.
7. Slowly descend and allow your heel to drop down slightly beneath the step or books before repeating.

Whilst these exercises may feel challenging, they should not increase heel pain or swelling. Do not continue with them if they do, and instead see your doctor for further advice.

Osteoarthritis

During the Covid pandemic I developed a grumbly knee. I put it down to my increased mileage outside walking, running and cycling, whilst gyms were closed and the country was in lockdown.

The patella (kneecap) functions to allow smooth movement as your knee bends or extends your leg. It does this by fitting into a groove at the end of your femur (thigh bone). Maltracking is where the patella isn't perfectly aligned with the groove. This can lead to cartilage loss, which in turn can lead to osteoarthritis.[5]

Over 10 million people in the UK are impacted by arthritis or other musculoskeletal conditions that affect joints. Of these, over 9 million are affected by the most common type of arthritis, osteoarthritis (OA). OA is a common joint disease. This is where the cartilage, which normally covers the end of bones within joints, degenerates. This damage compromises proper joint function, leading to inflammation, pain and restriction.

At present there is no way to prevent OA, although there are some known risk factors, which include:

- Age – more common in people over 45.
- Gender – greater prevalence in women, especially around menopause.
- Obesity – general wear and tear and damage to joints subject to increased weight-bearing forces.

- Inactivity – being sedentary reduces healthy joint function.
- Previous injury to joint.
- Genetics – some rarer forms of OA are thought to have a genetic link.

Women are more likely to be affected than men, the incidence of OA increases with age, and over a third of people aged between 45 and 75 seek treatment. OA typically affects the knees and hips, but other joints can be affected, including the spine, shoulders, elbows and hands. Over 4 million people aged over 45 years have OA of the knee, which is more common in women, and 2.9 million people aged over 45 have OA of the hip.

Exercise and knee issues

If you are a woman over 45 and you have niggly knees, you could have osteoarthritis. Even if you don't have osteoarthritis, but you have some level of restriction or discomfort in your knees, it's important to work on strength and stability. Strong supporting structures around your joints can significantly aid function and the ability to do the things you enjoy.

Before we get into some specific exercises it's helpful to understand how the knee moves. The knee is a hinge joint, opening and closing like a hinge on a door. Minimal rotation occurs in the knee, but it doesn't work in isolation; how your hips and feet are functioning can also affect the knee. The hips rotate and the complex structure of the foot means more movement happens here as well.

If there are movement restrictions in the hips and feet this can lead to compensation or greater forces in the knee joint. Working on hip and ankle mobility can be part of the solution when addressing many knee issues. In addition, when poor hip and ankle mobility are combined with repetitive movement the risk of injury or inflammation in the knee joint increases. This is why I have included lots of different exercises in different planes of movement, like side steps, reverse lunges and rotational jabs.

Test your ankle mobility

1. Do this exercise barefoot.
2. Adopt a kneeling lunge position on the floor, kneeling on your left leg, facing a wall. Put a cushion under your kneeling left knee for comfort, if needed. Use a measure to position your right foot and big toe exactly 12cm away from the wall.
3. Place your hands on the wall and lean in as you attempt to touch your right knee to the wall. Keep your right heel on the floor throughout.
4. Repeat the test on your left leg.
5. If your knee touches the wall, you have good mobility in your ankle. If your knee can't touch the wall, you have some restriction in your ankle mobility.

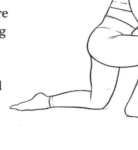

Test your hip mobility (the Thomas Test)

This test requires an elevated platform or surface on which you can safely and comfortably lie. One leg will be lowered over the edge during this test and your platform needs to be a sufficient height so that your foot does not touch the ground. A sturdy table with an

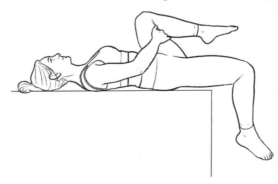

exercise mat on it, a high bed and mattress or a larger plyo box (commonly found in a gym setting used for plyometric exercises like box jumps) would all be suitable.

1. Lie on the elevated platform so that with your lower back is close to the edge.
2. Hug your knees to your chest.
3. Hold onto one of your knees whilst gently releasing your other leg.

Ideally, get someone to help you with this test by either taking a photograph sideways on, or describing what they can see.

> **Optimal** – *may indicate adequate hip mobility:* Able to pull knee fully to chest, back of lowered leg/butt remains in contact with the elevated platform, thigh of lowered leg is horizontal, hip, shoulder and knee joint aligned, 90-degree angle in knee of lowered leg.
>
> **Restricted** – *may indicate hip mobility restrictions:* Unable to pull knee to chest, back of lowered leg/butt lifts away from elevated platform, thigh of lowered leg is above horizontal, small amount of bend in the knee of lowered leg.[6]

The following exercises will help you work on hip mobility and ankle mobility.

90 90 hip stretch and 90 90 hip mobility

1. Do this exercise barefoot.
2. Sit on the floor with your knees bent at 90 degrees, feet flat on the floor.
3. Rotate your torso to your right, letting your knees travel to the right, keeping your feet in place.
4. The outside of your right leg, knee, ankle and foot, and the inside of your left leg, knee, ankle and foot should in contact with the floor so that you're sitting in a 90 90 position.
5. Inhale and relax into this stretch position as you exhale, put a cushion or Pilates block under your right knee for comfort if needed. Hold this stretch for up to 60 seconds.

6. To progress this stretch, try gently bringing your torso and chest forwards, towards your bent knees.
7. Rotate and bring your knees upwards and to the start position before swivelling them to the other side and repeating.

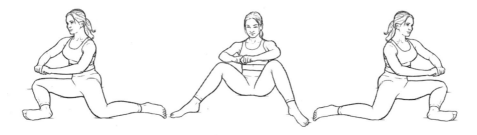

Half-kneeling ankle mobilisation

This is a similar set-up as the ankle mobility test but it incorporates dynamic movement to help you work on improving ankle mobility. Your foot and big toe will start closer to the wall than the ankle mobility test at first, though – 8cm rather than 12cm. As your ankle mobility improves over time, you'll move your foot and big toe further away from the wall.

1. Do this exercise barefoot.
2. Adopt a kneeling lunge position on the floor, kneeling on your left leg and facing a wall. Put a cushion under your kneeling left knee for comfort.
3. Use a measure to position your right foot and big toe exactly 8cm away from the wall.
4. Place your hands on the wall and lean in as you move your right knee towards the wall. Keep your right heel on the floor throughout.
5. Complete this exercise slowly to a count of 5, relax and repeat several times.
6. Change sides.

As your ankle flexibility improves, and once your knee can touch the wall, place your foot further away from the wall for this mobilisation exercise.

The following exercises can assist with knee stability and maintain strength in your quads.

Lying straight leg raises
Sets: 2   **Reps:** 8–12
1. Lie on your back, resting your arms at your sides.
2. Bend your right knee with your foot flat on the floor, keep your left leg extended, with a flexed foot.
3. Inhale, and on the exhale gently lift your left leg upwards so your foot is about 30–40cm away from the floor.
4. Lower with control.
5. Repeat on the other side.

Single leg squat touchdown
Sets: 2   **Reps:** 8–12
1. Use a low step or put a couple of thick sturdy books on the floor.
2. Stand on the low step or books on your right leg.
3. Take your left leg slightly to the side with a flexed foot.
4. Push the hips back, bending at the knee, and allow the chest to come forwards. Do not allow your right knee to travel forwards, keep it over the ankle.
5. Tap down to the floor with your left heel before straightening your right leg back to the start position.

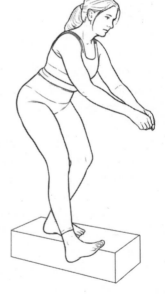

Wall sits
Sets: 1   **Hold:** 20–30 seconds
1. Stand facing away from a wall, with your feet hip distance apart, about 60cm away from the wall.
2. Lean your back towards the wall.
3. Slide and lower your bottom downwards so the whole of your back is in contact with the wall, to a depth you can comfortably hold – anywhere between 40 and 90 degrees.

If any of these exercises cause pain, please stop and seek further advice from your doctor.

Adhesive capsulitis (frozen shoulder)

Adhesive capsulitis, commonly known as frozen shoulder, has an estimated incidence of 2–5 per cent and affects as many as one in 10 women – commonly around menopause. The condition causes stiffness and pain in the shoulder joint, and severely limits movement. The pain can be especially bad at night, and many women with adhesive capsulitis will find their sleep is severely impacted as a result. The condition can last months and often years.

Most women will not require surgery to resolve this condition. Unfortunately, no amount of rest, physio, stretching and mobility work made an iota of difference in my case, so eventually my consultant recommended a surgical procedure known as arthroscopic capsular release and decompression. This involves releasing the tight capsule around the shoulder and sometimes removing scarring and part of the capsule.

What causes the development of adhesive capsulitis is not currently known, although it is thought there could be a connection between the loss of oestrogen in menopause and the condition. In one study it has been shown that the use of hormonal treatment therapy appears to reduce the risk of shoulder pain.[7]

At present there are no known ways to prevent the development of a frozen shoulder, and if you have already experienced the condition in one shoulder you are at an increased risk of developing it in your other shoulder.

Whether you do or don't have experience of frozen shoulder (or other shoulder issues), maintaining functional movement and strength can become harder with increasing age. Gravity and lifestyle factors, like working on a PC, driving and scrolling on your phone, can all affect posture. Medical conditions like osteoporosis and ageing of the spine and discs also impacts posture. Muscles around the front of the shoulder can become tight and restricted, resulting in a rounded shoulders appearance.

The following exercises are valuable and may help improve range of movement if you have restrictions in your shoulders, and they are also useful for the maintenance of shoulder health, along with the shoulder-strengthening exercises in Chapter 8.

If you currently have frozen shoulder, please consult with your doctor before attempting these exercises.

Frozen shoulder exercises

These exercises are best repeated often and throughout the day if you are struggling with a frozen shoulder. They can be helpful in both easing discomfort and assisting with a range of movement.

Pendulum swings

Sets: 1   Reps: 8–12
1. Rest the palm of your unaffected arm on a table and let your affected arm hang down loosely.
2. Gently move your body a little to initiate small swings in your arm.
3. Try circular movements in both directions as well.

Assisted arm pullover

Sets: 1   Reps: 8–12
1. Lie on your back, palms resting on your thighs.
2. With the hand from your unaffected arm, clasp the wrist of your affected arm.
3. Raise your affected arm up and over your head as far as you can comfortably go, using your unaffected arm to assist.
4. Hold for up to 10 seconds and return to the start.

Seated shoulder stretch

Sets: 1   **Hold:** 10–30 seconds

1. Hold a towel or resistance band in the hand of your unaffected arm.
2. Raise your arm upwards, bend at the elbow, and drop the towel or band down behind your back.
3. Take your affected arm behind your back, bending at the elbow, and hold the other end of the towel or band with this hand.
4. Use the hand of your unaffected arm to gently pull the towel or band upwards whilst increasing the stretch in your affected shoulder.

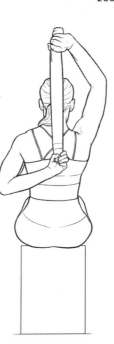

Daily shoulder health exercises

Lifestyle factors like time spent scrolling on mobile phones, desk-based jobs, working on a computer and driving can all affect shoulder alignment and posture. The following exercises are useful as part of a shoulder health maintenance programme. You don't have to be experiencing shoulder issues to benefit from them.

Side lying external rotation

Sets: 1   **Reps:** 8–12

1. Lie on your left-hand side, resting your head on a cushion or your forearm.

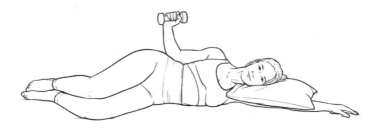

2. Hold a very light dumbbell or water bottle in your right hand.
3. Keep your upper arm fixed to your body and bent at the elbow.
4. With your palm facing downwards, gently raise and rotate your arm, maintaining a 90-degree angle at your elbow.
5. Slowly lower and return to the start.

From the additional floor-based dynamic mobility exercises on page 152.
Sets: 1   Reps: 6–8

Floor angel

1. Lie on your back, then bend both knees, keeping the feet flat on the floor.
2. Rest your arms on the floor above your head.
3. Bend your elbows to a right angle and in line with your shoulders, palms up.
4. Slide your elbows down, slightly pressing them into the floor to make a 'V' shape with your body.
5. Now slide your elbows upwards, maintaining a 'V' shape between your upper arm and forearm.
6. Bring your fingertips together over your head as you slide your arms upwards.
7. Slide your elbows downwards again.

From the resistance band strength exercises on page 192.

Pulldown

1. From a standing position, hold onto the resistance band, wrapping each end around each of your palms until your hands are slightly wider than shoulder distance apart.
2. Extend your arms up overhead vertically.
3. Pull each end of the band in an arc either side of your body so that your arms are parallel to the floor and in line with your shoulders.
4. Return to the start position.

Pull apart

1. From a standing position, hold onto the resistance band, wrapping each end around each of your palms until your hands are slightly wider than shoulder distance apart.
2. Extend and lift your arms upwards to shoulder height, palms facing each other.
3. Pull the band apart and your palms away from one another until your arms are fully extended on either side of your body in a 'T' shape.
4. Return to the start position.

Y T A

1. Holding each end of the resistance band in each hand, anchor the middle of the band at mid-chest height, then face the anchor point and step backwards.
2. Extend and lift your arms upwards to shoulder height, palms facing each other. This is your start position.
3. Keeping your arms extended, with thumbs and handles rotated away from the body, lift them overhead and outwards at an angle into a 'Y' shape.
4. Return to the start position before lowering your extended arms to the sides of your body in a 'T' shape.
5. Return to the start position before extending your arms and lowering them outwards at an angle into an 'A' shape.
6. Return to the start position.

I hope this chapter gives you hope, and if you are challenged with a musculoskeletal issue remember the golden rule – assess don't guess. Once you know what you are dealing with you can make some informed decisions on how to manage this, and how to exercise and work around this.

CHAPTER 13

STRETCH IT OUT

I'm a firm believer that how you start your day sets the tone for the day. Likewise, unwinding and relaxing at the end of the day is valuable and can aid restful sleep.

My mornings typically start with a sunrise walk, run or cycle on the beach where I live. Apart from the benefit of starting the day with some cardiovascular, heart-healthy exercise, exposure to early morning sunlight is known to positively influence circadian rhythm, sleep and mood.[1]

You don't have to get up at sunrise and work out first thing in the morning if it doesn't suit you or your schedule. Instead, you can still benefit from exposure to natural daylight and a short stretching session to ease any morning muscle stiffness, aid circulation and start your day energised – whatever time you rise!

Try to stand, sit or walk outside, even if it's no more than 10 minutes, as soon as possible on waking. Couple this with drinking a large glass of water, which will help rehydrate your body after sleep. Morning sunlight helps signal to your body and your circadian rhythm what time it is and influences your sleep cycle and hormone production.

Follow this with my brief morning mobility and stretch routine, which starts on the floor and brings you to standing by the end, leaving you ready for the day.

Morning mobility and stretching

From the additional floor-based dynamic mobility exercises, page 152.
Reps: 6–8

Cat cow
1. Start in an all-fours position.
2. Exhale as you round the spine upwards, tucking the head and pelvis downwards.
3. Inhale, release the back to the start position and continue in a flowing movement, allowing your belly to drop downwards.
4. Lift your head and neck, and your pelvis upwards as your spine curves downwards.

Half-kneeling lunge to hamstring stretch
1. Start in a lunge position, kneeling on your left knee and extending your right leg, bending at the knee and with your foot on the ground. Both knees should now be at 90 degrees.
2. Push the hips backwards, allowing your right leg to extend, and reach your hands forward towards your right foot.
3. Now reverse the movement, this time lifting your arms up overhead and pushing your hips further forwards.
4. Repeat on the other side.

From stretches for the whole body on page 205.
Hold: 15–20 seconds

Child's pose
1. Kneel on all fours, then sit back on your heels, opening your thighs wider as you do so.
2. Stretch your arms and upper body out in front of you.
3. Sink your upper body between your open thighs, with palms flat on the floor.

Thread the needle
1. Knee on all fours.
2. Sit back on your heels, opening your thighs wider as you do so.
3. Stretch your arms and upper body out in front of you.
4. Exhale and bring your right arm underneath your left arm and shoulder with your palm facing upwards.
5. Rest the right side of your face on your exercise mat and look towards your outstretched right arm and hand.

6. Hold for 15–20 seconds before pushing back to all fours and changing sides.

From the whole-body warm-up activity on page 148.
Reps: 6–8

Shoulders
1. Lift your shoulders up to your ears, then roll them backwards and down.
2. Make the movement bigger by circling the arms as you roll the shoulders, extending and raising your arms to the front and up – overhead, backwards and downwards.
3. Reverse the movement by lifting the arms backwards and up overhead, before circling forwards and downwards again.
4. Now alternate the arms in a backward crawl, swimming-type movement.
5. Repeat to the front in a front-crawl swimming-type movement.

Abdominals, back and shoulders
1. Widen your stance.
2. Reach your hands upwards and across your body in a diagonal movement to your right, allowing your left heel to lift off the floor as you rotate through your torso, and feel the weight shift to your right leg.
3. Lengthen through your back at the same time so that your arms are outstretched from the top of your fingertips on your right hand, through to the toes on your left foot.
4. Now imagine you are tracing an upside-down rainbow as your hands lead the movement, arcing downwards and then upwards to your left-hand side.
5. As you do this your left heel returns to the floor, so your left foot is balanced and flat and your right heel lifts upwards as you pivot on the toes of your right foot.
6. Repeat this sweeping arc movement, aiming to rotate a little more with each repetition.

From the pulse-lowering exercises on page 201.
Reps: 3

Standing reach to semi-squat with fingertip sweep

1. Stand with feet hip distance apart.
2. Raise your arms up overhead and rise onto your toes at the same time (if possible).
3. While performing a semi-squat movement – hinging at the hip and bending at the knees – flow your arms back downwards, keeping them straight, and try to sweep the floor with your fingertips.
4. Repeat, keeping the movement slow and gentle.

Just as a morning mobility routine can set us up for the day, an evening stretch and relax can help us leave any stress of the day behind and aid restful sleep.

The routine starts from a standing position and is designed to flow effortlessly from one stretch or mobility exercise to the next, until you finish in a lying position. You could even complete the whole routine in your pyjamas and finish the final two stretches in your bed and allow yourself to drift off to sleep!

Evening stretch and relaxation

This evening stretch and relaxation routine takes just a few minutes to complete. It can help release any build-up of tension you have accumulated during the day, ease off muscle stiffness and set you up for a restful night's sleep.

Roll down from standing

1. Stand with your feet hip distance apart.
2. Let your arms stay loose and relaxed at your sides.
3. Inhale, then with your next exhale, starting from the top of your head, gently and slowly roll your spine downwards.

4. Maintain soft knees until your fingertips touch the ground or you have reached as far as is comfortable for you.
5. Inhale as you start to roll gently back to the top, re-stacking your vertebrae from the base of your spine to the top of your neck and head.
6. Repeat 4–5 times.
7. As you reach the downward phase of your final repetition, bend and sink to your knees whilst walking your hands forwards until you are in an all-fours position.
8. Flow into child's pose.
9. Kneel on all fours, then sit back on your heels, opening your thighs wider as you do so.
10. Stretch your arms and upper body out in front of you.
11. Sink your upper body between your open thighs with palms flat on the floor and hold for 20–30 seconds.
12. Flow back to all-fours, then into a half-kneeling position and continue with a half-kneeling lunge to hamstring stretch.
13. Start in a lunge position, kneeling on your left knee and extending your right leg, bending at the knee, foot on the ground. Both knees should now be at 90 degrees.
14. Push the hips backwards, allowing your right leg to extend, and reach your hands forward towards your right foot.
15. Now reverse the movement, this time lifting your arms up overhead, and pushing your hips further forwards. Repeat 5 times and change sides.
16. Flow from the half-kneeling position to a seated position to continue with the seated lateral neck stretch.
17. Sit with a neutral spine posture, hands rested at your sides. Looking straight ahead, gently tilt your head sideways to the right.
18. Decrease the distance between your right ear and right shoulder, keeping your shoulders straight and level throughout.
19. Assist the stretch by bringing your right arm over your head and cradling the left-hand side of your head with your right hand. Apply gentle pressure and hold for 20–30 seconds.
20. Change sides and repeat.

To flow from seated to lying
Sitting with legs extended to the front, knees bent with feet flat on the floor, hold on to the back of your thighs. Gently roll down from the base of your spine until your back is completely flat on the floor.

Continue with lying thoracic rotation stretch
1. Lie on your back, arms outstretched and palms upwards to make a 'T' shape with your body.
2. Bend your right knee and cross your right foot over your left knee, resting it on the floor.
3. Rest your left hand on the side of your right knee and apply gentle pressure.
4. Turn your head to the right to look at your outstretched right arm. Hold for 20–30 seconds.
5. Repeat on the other side.
6. Remain on your back for the final stretch and some relaxed and calm breathing.

Whole-body stretch
1. Lie on your back with your arms relaxed at your sides, palms up and legs extended and straight.
2. Inhale, and on the exhale focus on releasing any tension and imagine melting into the mat.
3. Relax your abdominal muscles.
4. Close your eyes (if this feels comfortable for you) and bring your focus to your breathing.
5. Remain in this whole-body stretch for 1–2 minutes.

CHAPTER 14

DEMYSTIFYING EXERCISE

All professions, interests and groups develop their own terminology. These terms can sound confusing to anyone on the outside, and fitness is no different; lots of terms, words, phrases and abbreviations are used. It has been my intention to simplify language and make this book user-friendly and accessible wherever possible, but at the same time, I think it's helpful to be familiar with the more commonly used fitness terms. This exercise glossary contains those you are most likely to come across.

Active recovery – low-intensity exercise on a day that usually follows a more intense form of exercise performed on the previous day. It can be more beneficial to the body than complete rest as it aids blood flow, waste removal and muscle recovery after strenuous exercise. Walking, swimming and cycling are all examples of activities that support active recovery.

Aerobic exercise – physical activity that elevates the heart rate and increases the body's use of oxygen. Oxygen is required to fuel any physical activity with a duration of over 2 minutes. Aerobic exercise is also known as cardiovascular exercise.

Anaerobic exercise – intense physical activity that's shorter in duration than aerobic exercise. These short bouts of high-intensity exercise last anywhere between 10 and 90 seconds. Glucose in the body is broken down to use as fuel, rather than oxygen.

Beats per minute (bpm) – the number of beats the heart makes in a minute.

Cardiovascular exercise – activity that elevates the heart rate and increases the body's use of oxygen. Oxygen is required to fuel any physical activity with a duration of over 2 minutes. Cardiovascular exercise is also known as aerobic exercise.

Circuit training – several different exercises, often referred to as stations, that are performed one after the other. Together, these are known as a circuit. Once every exercise in the circuit is complete, a period of rest may follow before the circuit is repeated. Exercises in a circuit can be performed with body weight, small training tools or weights. Circuit training typically includes a mixture of resistance, cardiovascular and core exercises, but it can also focus on one component of fitness.

Compound exercise – an exercise that involves multiple muscle groups, over several joints, at the same time. These exercises often require more skill, energy and proficiency to perform than those for smaller muscle groups. Consequently, compound exercises are usually the first exercises in a training programme. A deadlift is an example of a compound exercise, as it is a demanding whole-body exercise.

Cooldown – a period of recovery after a workout that allows the body to recover and the heart rate to return to normal. A specific cooldown should be tailored to the main session. A cooldown following cardiovascular exercise will include a pulse-lowering activity and stretching. Cooldowns following other activities may include stretching and relaxation.

Core – a group of muscles in the mid-section that stabilise the spine. These include the abdominal, back and pelvic muscles.

Core training – exercises that strengthen and condition the core muscles.

Cross-training – training with different types of movement and exercises. Cross-training is a rounded approach, with the aim of achieving skill or competency across many components of fitness.

DOMS – delayed onset muscle soreness. This refers to the muscle stiffness and soreness that can follow activity in the first 24–48 hours afterwards. It is a normal response to exercise that is new, strenuous or particularly challenging. It indicates temporary inflammation and microscopic damage to muscle fibres. The adaptive process of muscle fibres means they get stronger as a result. Which is why you won't always experience DOMS with the same exercise once you are accustomed to it. Blood flow to the area is necessary to reduce inflammation and repair any damage, which is why active recovery is helpful.

Dynamic warm-up – this involves a series of movements, taking joints and muscles through a full range of movement. It involves dynamic stretching as the muscles are not held in a lengthened state during the warm-up, but both lengthen and contract during the movements. A dynamic warm-up helps raise core temperature and blood flow to the working muscles in preparation for the exercise that follows.

Endurance exercise – exercise over an extended period of time that requires cardiovascular endurance and muscular endurance. A marathon is an example of an endurance form of exercise.

Frequency – refers to how often a specific exercise or session takes place.

Functional exercise or movement – any exercise or movement that either improves or maintains the functions of the body, joints and muscles to move in a variety of ways. This can include pushing, pulling, rotating, lifting, twisting, forwards, backwards and sideways movement. Functional exercise may be aimed at supporting a specific activity of daily life – such as squats to help promote sitting down into a chair and getting back up again. It can also be useful for athletic performance.

Heart rate (HR) – the number of times the heart beats, normally within 60 seconds.

Heart rate zones – normally calculated as different percentages based on maximum heart rate. Referring to heart rate training zones can clarify the level of intensity you are working at.

HIIT – high intensity interval training. A training protocol where short bursts of high intensity are followed by a period of rest. The intensity of a HIIT workout means it is usually carried out over a short period of between 20 and 40 minutes. A popular work-to-rest ratio is often 1:1 or 1:2 for cardiovascular fitness – for example, 30 seconds of work followed by up to 30 seconds' rest. When working on explosive power a longer rest period may be required, such as 1:5 – for example, 15 seconds of work followed by 75 seconds' rest.

Interval training – a series of repeated rounds of exercise where work periods are alternated with rest periods.

Isolation exercise – an exercise where a muscle group is worked in isolation, and where no more than one joint is involved. A biceps curl is an example of an isolation exercise.

Isometric exercise – exercise where a static contraction of muscle occurs, but without movement in a joint or muscle. A plank hold is an example of an isometric exercise.

Maximum heart rate (MHR) – the highest number, and upper limit, of how many times your heart can beat in a minute under stress.

Plyometric exercise – a type of training that involves speed and force to build muscle power. Ball slams are an example of an upper body plyometric exercise.

Posterior chain – all the muscles and structures at the back of your body are known collectively as the posterior chain. It includes some of the largest muscle groups of the body. An example of an exercise that recruits numerous muscles of the posterior chain is a deadlift.

Progressive overload – is a principal of resistance training. It's where muscles are incrementally overloaded, over time, which causes the muscles to adapt and get bigger and/or stronger.

Reps – repetitions. The number of complete movements of an exercise.

Resistance training – a type of physical activity where the body is required to resist a weight or force. This can lead to an increase in muscle size, strength, power and endurance. Also known as strength training and weight training.

Rest – a defined period of recovery that follows a work period. This can be applied to strength training and interval workouts.

Resting heart rate (RHR) – the number of times the heart beats at rest.

RPE – rate of perceived exertion. A technique to gauge exercise intensity based on self-assessment.

Sets – a collection of reps.

Strength training – a type of physical activity where the body is required to resist a weight or force. This can lead to an increase in muscle size, strength, power and endurance. Also known as resistance training and weight training.

Tempo – the rate, pace or speed at which a repetition with a weight, or a body-weight exercise is performed. An example of a tempo in strength training is 3:3, which would be 3 seconds for the push or pull phase of a movement and 3 seconds to return to the start position. A tempo can also include a pause, for example, a chest press could be 3:1:3, which means 3 seconds as the dumbbells are lowered, 1 second pause at the bottom of the movement, then 3 seconds to push upwards.

Unilateral exercise – an exercise where only one side or one limb is dominant in the movement. A single arm shoulder press is an example of a unilateral exercise.

Weight training – a type of physical activity where the body is required to resist a weight or force. This can lead to an increase in muscle size, strength, power and endurance. Also known as resistance training and strength training.

Muscle groups

There are over 600 muscles in the human body. Muscle names are often hard to remember, as they derive from Greek and Latin, and you don't need to know all of them. However, it's helpful to be familiar with the main muscles that are frequently referred to in exercise and fitness, and where they can be found on the body.

Abs – abbreviation of abdominal muscles.
Biceps – a muscle at the front of the upper arm that runs from the shoulder to the elbow.
Calves – muscles in the back of the lower leg.
Deltoids – a large triangular muscle that covers the shoulders.
Glutes – a group of muscles in the buttocks.
Hamstrings – muscles at the back of the thigh.
Lats – a broad, flat muscle of the middle and lower back.
Pecs – muscles in the chest.
Quads – muscles at the front of the thigh.
Triceps – a muscle at the back of the upper arm.

FINAL THOUGHTS

I have always believed it's a privilege to grow old. The older I become, the more I appreciate this truism. I have outlived friends, clients and colleagues whose lives were cut short by illness, accident and, sadly, death by suicide. I have lived the life my brother Jonathon was denied, I've enjoyed the things he never got around to doing – career highs, travelling, getting married, having children and grandchildren, and writing this, my first book, and seeing it published!

We are lucky if we make it, but we don't have to rely on luck when it comes to healthier ageing. What you do from this day onwards has the power to influence your future health trajectory, and what the final 10–15 years of your life will be like. It has the potential power to make the difference between living and simply existing. You don't need motivation, you simply need to make physical activity a non-negotiable part of your life, for the rest of your life. Let it become a habit that's second nature to you, like brushing your teeth every day.

This book has provided you with a roadmap, a way to navigate ageing and avoid some of the pitfalls like sedentary behaviour and poor nutrition, to arrive at your final destination and declare, 'What a wonderful journey this has been!'

ACKNOWLEDGEMENTS

When my publisher, Katya Shipster from HarperCollins, contacted me in September 2022 to ask if I'd be interested in writing a book, I was excited and terrified in equal measures. Writing a non-fiction book is a big undertaking. The importance of including accurate and evidence-based information is a responsibility I haven't taken lightly. Katya I'm incredibly grateful to you for believing in my ability to do this book justice. Your expert guidance, along with Julia and George, has shaped it into something I'm enormously proud of.

Jan and the team at DML, Borra, Lou and Megan, from our first meeting when you asked if I'd ever thought about writing a book, I have felt supported and in safe hands. Thank you for nurturing my career and always having my best interests at heart.

Drawing on knowledge from an amazing team of experts Dr Nighat Arif, Dr Charlotte Ord, Dr Jenna Macciochi, Clare Bourne and Priya Tew, has enabled me to expand on important topics in this book. I'm very grateful for their time in answering my many questions.

Fit and fearless females who epitomise active ageing, Carol Norris and Sheila Nollert, thank you for sharing your amazing stories with me. No doubt other women will feel inspired to embark on their own challenges after reading about yours.

A physically active lifestyle reduces, but doesn't eliminate, the risk of developing some diseases. Mary Huckle was an inspirational woman who campaigned relentlessly for better funding and research into metastatic breast cancer. Thank you to Mary's family for allowing me to share her story and honour her memory.

My parents, who are in their eighties, are wonderful examples of ageing joyfully, despite some of the challenges older age can bring. I love you more than words could ever say, thank you for being the most supportive parents I could have asked for.

Chris, you'd think after 40 years of marriage we could make each other a cup of tea that's drinkable! We may have different opinions on the perfect brew but, tea making skills aside, I truly appreciate you being the rock I can always depend on.

My five beautiful and brilliant children Tobias, Poppy, Gabriel, Saffron and Jasper, you have always been my reason why. Saffron, as the other published author in the family, I am so grateful for all your writerly tips!

To Mazen, Chloe and the team at Women's Best, thank you for supplying me with stunning sportswear and my cover look for this book.

Finally, without my Instagram online community and clients, this book might never have come about. You have been instrumental in moulding me into a better trainer, coach and active ageing advocate. Thank you, this book is for you.

ENDNOTES

MY FITNESS JOURNEY

1. Lee M. and Carroll T.J., 'Cross education: Possible mechanisms for the contralateral effects of unilateral resistance training', *Sports Medicine*, 2007. (https://pubmed.ncbi.nlm.nih.gov/17190532/)

CHAPTER 1

1. Xue, Shanshan, et al, 'Age at attainment of peak bone mineral density and its associated factors: The National Health and Nutrition Examination Survey 2005–2014', 21 November 2019. (https://pubmed.ncbi.nlm.nih.gov/31760214/)
2. Ji, Meng-Xia and Yu, Qi, 'Primary osteoporosis in postmenopausal women', *Chronic Diseases & Translational Medicine*, 21 March 2015. (www.ncbi.nlm.nih.gov/pmc/articles/PMC5643776/#bib12)
3. The International Osteoporosis Foundation. (www.osteoporosis. foundation/health-professionals/about-osteoporosis/epidemiology)
4. Arena, Ross, et al, 'Revisiting age-predicted maximal heart rate: Can it be used as a valid measure of effort?' *Am Heart J,* 17 December 2015. (www.ncbi.nlm.nih.gov/pmc/articles/PMC4919019/)
5. Gulati, Martha, et al, 'Heart rate response to exercise stress testing in asymptomatic women', *Circulation,* 28 June 2010. (www.ahajournals. org/doi/10.1161/CIRCULATIONAHA.110.939249)
6. Alway, S.E., et al, 'Contrasts in muscle and myofibers of elite male and female bodybuilders', *Journal of Applied Physiology*, 1 July 1989. (https:// journals.physiology.org/doi/abs/10.1152/jappl.1989.67.1.24)
7. Clark, Brian C. and Manini, Todd M., 'Sarcopenia ≠ Dynapenia', *The Journals of Gerontology: Series A*, 8 August 2008. (https://academic.oup. com/biomedgerontology/article/63/8/829/567368?login=false)

8. Volpi, Elena, et al, 'Muscle tissue changes with aging', *Curr Opin Clin Nutr Metab Care*, 12 January 2010. (www.ncbi.nlm.nih.gov/pmc/articles/PMC2804956/)

9. Sheppard, J.M. and Young, W.B., 'Agility literature review: Classifications, training and testing', *Journal of Sports Science*, September 2006. (https://pubmed.ncbi.nlm.nih.gov/16882626/)

10. El-Khoury, Fabienne, et al, 'The effect of fall prevention exercise programmes on fall induced injuries in community dwelling older adults: Systematic review and meta-analysis of randomised controlled trials', *British Medical Journal*, 29 October 2013. (www.bmj.com/content/347/bmj.f6234)

11. Hardwick, Robert M., et al, 'Age-related increases in reaction time result from slower preparation, not delayed initiation', *Journal of Neurophysiology*, 13 July 2022. (https://pubmed.ncbi.nlm.nih.gov/35829640/)

12. Mahase, Elisabeth, 'Stop using body mass index as measure of health, say MPs', *British Medical Journal*, 9 April 2021. (www.bmj.com/content/373/bmj.n941)

13. 'Waist circumference and waist-hip ratio: Report of a WHO expert consultation', World Health Organization, 8–11 December 2008. (www.who.int/publications/i/item/9789241501491)

14. Brian Mac Sports Coach. (https://www.brianmac.co.uk/vo2max.htm)

15. Kline, G.M., et al, 'Estimation of VO2max from a one-mile track walk, gender, age, and body weight', *Medicine and Science in Sports and Exercise*, July 1987. (www.researchgate.net/publication/19562170_Estimation_of_VO2max_from_a_one-mile_track_walk_gender_age_and_body_weight)

16. Heywood, V. (2006) *The Physical Fitness Specialist Manual*, The Cooper Institute for Aerobics Research, Dallas TX, Advanced Fitness Assessment and Exercise Prescription, Fifth Edition, Champaign, IL: Human Kinetics.

17. Body-weight squat assessment protocol. (https://acewebcontent.azureedge.net/assets/certification/ace-answers/forms/pt/37_Bodyweight_Squat_Assessment_Protocol.pdf)

18. American College of Sports Medicine Guidelines for Exercise Testing and Prescription. (www.acsm.org/education-resources/books/guidelines-exercise-testing-prescription)

19. 'In brief: How does our sense of balance work?', *Institute for Quality and Efficiency in Health Care,* last updated 25 September 2023. (www.ncbi.nlm.nih.gov/books/NBK279394/)

20. Gil Araujo, Claudio, et al, 'Successful 10-second one-legged stance performance predicts survival in middle-aged and older individuals', *British Journal of Sports Medicine.* (https://bjsm.bmj.com/content/56/17/975)

21. Physical activity guidelines: UK Chief Medical Officers' report, UK Government, 7 September 2019. (www.gov.uk/government/publications/physical-activity-guidelines-uk-chief-medical-officers-report)

22. 'Physical Activity', World Health Organization, 26 June 2024. (www.who.int/news-room/fact-sheets/detail/physical-activity)

CHAPTER 2

1. Winchester, Nicole, 'Women's health outcomes: Is there a gender gap?', House of Lords Library, 1 July 2021. (https://lordslibrary.parliament.uk/womens-health-outcomes-is-there-a-gender-gap/)

2. 'Women with dementia receive less medical attention', UCL News, 5 December 2016. (www.ucl.ac.uk/news/2016/dec/women-dementia-receive-less-medical-attention)

3. Zimmermann, Martina, et al, 'Shifting how we view the ageing process', King's College London, 2023. (https://kclpure.kcl.ac.uk/portal/en/publications/shifting-how-we-view-the-ageing-process)

4. Mitina, Maria, et al, 'Psychological aging, depression, and well-being', *Aging* (Albany NY), 18 September 2020. (www.ncbi.nlm.nih.gov/pmc/articles/PMC7585090/)

5. Diehl, Manfred, et al, 'Awareness of aging: Theoretical considerations on an emerging concept', *Developmental Review,* June 2014. (www.sciencedirect.com/science/article/abs/pii/S0273229714000021)

6. Charles, Susan and Carstensen, Laura L., 'Social and emotional aging', *Annual Review of Psychology,* 12 March 2014. (www.ncbi.nlm.nih.gov/pmc/articles/PMC3950961/)

7. 'The concept and experience of aging' (https://courses.lumenlearning.com/suny-socialproblems/chapter/6-1-the-concept-and-experience-of-aging/)

8. WHO/HPS Geneva 2000

9. 'Health state life expectancies, UK: 2018 to 2020, Census, 4 March 2022. (www.ons.gov.uk/peoplepopulationandcommunity/health andsocialcare/healthandlifeexpectancies/bulletins/healthstatelife expectanciesuk/2018to2020)

10. National life tables – life expectancy in the UK: 2020 to 2022, UK government, 11 January 2024. (www.ons.gov.uk/peoplepopulation andcommunity/birthsdeathsandmarriages/lifeexpectancies/ bulletins/nationallifetablesunitedkingdom/2020to2022)

11. Guo, Hui Jun and Sapra, Amit, 'Instrumental activity of daily living', *StatPearls*, 14 November 2022. (www.ncbi.nlm.nih.gov/books/ NBK553126/)

12. Clark, D., 'Life expectancy at birth in the United Kingdom from 2018 to 2020, by gender and local area', 1 October 2024. (www.statista.com/ statistics/296698/local-areas-with-highest-male-life-expectancy -united-kingdom-uk/)

13. Burd, Nicholas A., et al, 'Anabolic resistance of muscle protein synthesis with aging', *Exercise and Sport Sciences Reviews*, July 2013. (https://journals.lww.com/acsm-essr/fulltext/2013/07000/anabolic_ resistance_of_muscle_protein_synthesis.6.aspx)

14. Finkelstein, Joel S., et al, 'Bone mineral density changes during the menopause transition in a multiethnic cohort of women', *Journal of Clinical Endocrinology and Metabolism*, 26 December 2007. (www.ncbi. nlm.nih.gov/pmc/articles/PMC2266953/)

15. 'Bone mineral density decreases less than expected after menopause', University of Eastern Finland, 27 October 2021. (www.sciencedaily. com/releases/2021/10/211027122047.htm)

16. Clausen, Johan S.R., et al, 'Midlife cardiorespiratory fitness and the long-term risk of mortality', *Journal of the American College of Cardiology*, 2018. (www.jacc.org/doi/epdf/10.1016/j.jacc.2018.06.045)

17. Stathokostas, Liza, et al, 'Flexibility of older adults aged 55–86 years and the influence of physical activity', *Journal of Aging Research*, 19 June 2013. (www.ncbi.nlm.nih.gov/pmc/articles/PMC3703899/)

18. 'Ageing: Ageism', World Health Organization, 18 March 2021. (www. who.int/news-room/questions-and-answers/item/ageing-ageism)

19. Brinkhof, Lotte P., et al 'The Subjective Experience of Ageism: The Perceived Ageism Questionnaire (PAQ)', *International Journal of Environmental Research and Public Health*, 19 July 2022. (www.ncbi.nlm. nih.gov/pmc/articles/PMC9319588/#B11-ijerph-19-08792)

20. Levy, Becca R., et al, 'Longevity increased by positive self-perceptions of aging', *Journal of Personal & Social Psychology*, August 2002. (https://pubmed.ncbi.nlm.nih.gov/12150226/)

21. Passarino, Giuseppe, et al, 'Human longevity: Genetics or lifestyle? It takes two to tango', *Immunity and Ageing*, 5 April 2016. (www.ncbi.nlm.nih.gov/pmc/articles/PMC4822264/)

CHAPTER 3

1. UK Chief Medical Officers' Physical Activity Guidelines, 2019; London: Department of Health and Social Care.

2. Physical activity: applying All Our Health, Public Health England, 10 March 2022. (www.gov.uk/government/publications/physical-activity-applying-all-our-health/physical-activity-applying-all-our-health)

3. Health Survey for England – 2012, NHS England, 18 December 2013. (https://digital.nhs.uk/data-and-information/publications/statistical/health-survey-for-england/health-survey-for-england-2012)

4. Physical Activity, World Health Organization, 26 June 2024. (www.who.int/news-room/fact-sheets/detail/physical-activity)

5. Met Up UK. (https://metupuk.org.uk/)

6. Carol Norris. (www.instagram.com/tournesol_fitness_with_carol/)

7. Grandma Moves. (www.instagram.com/grandma_moves/)

8. 'Fear of injury preventing over 55s benefiting from exercise', Nuffield Health. (www.nuffieldhealth.com/article/fear-of-injury-preventing-over-55s-benefiting-from-exercise)

9. Anderson, Elizabeth and Durstine, J. Larry, 'Physical activity, exercise, and chronic diseases: A brief review', *Sports Medicine and Health Science*, 10 September 2019. (www.ncbi.nlm.nih.gov/pmc/articles/PMC9219321/)

10. Physical activity, World Health Organization, 26 June 2024. (www.who.int/news-room/fact-sheets/detail/physical-activity)

11. Physical activity: applying All Our Health, Public Health England, 10 March 2022. (www.gov.uk/government/publications/physical-activity-applying-all-our-health/physical-activity-applying-all-our-health)

12. Moreno-Agostino, Darío, et al, 'The impact of physical activity on healthy ageing trajectories: evidence from eight cohort studies', *International Journal of Behavioral Nutrition and Physical Activity*, 16 July 2020. (https://ijbnpa.biomedcentral.com/articles/10.1186/s12966-020-00995-8)

CHAPTER 4

1. 'Changing the future of women's health', Women's Health Initiative. (www.whi.org/)
2. Bluming, Avrum Z., et al, "Tis but a scratch: a critical review of the Women's Health Initiative evidence associating menopausal hormone therapy with the risk of breast cancer', *Menopause, The Journal of the Menopause Society*, December 2023. (https://journals.lww.com/ menopausejournal/abstract/2023/12000/_tis_but_a_scratch__a_ critical_review_of_the.10.aspx)
3. 'Menopause: diagnosis and management', NICE Guidelines, 5 December 2019. (www.nice.org.uk/guidance/ng23)
4. 'Leading charity urges action as analysis shows dementia has been UK women's leading cause of death for a decade', *Alzheimer's Research* UK, 15 May 2022. (www.alzheimersresearchuk.org/news/leading-charity -urges-action-as-analysis-shows-dementia-has-been-uk-womens -leading-cause-of-death-for-a-decade/)
5. Erickson, Kirk I., et al, 'Exercise training increases size of hippocampus and improves memory', *Proceedings of the National Academy of Sciences USA*, 31 August 2011. (www.ncbi.nlm.nih.gov/pmc/articles/PMC3041121/)
6. Tan, Zaldy S., et al, 'Physical activity, brain volume, and dementia risk: The Framingham Study', *The Journals of Gerontology*, 15 July 2016. (www.ncbi.nlm.nih.gov/pmc/articles/PMC6075525/)
7. Gheysen, Freja, et al, 'Physical activity to improve cognition in older adults: can physical activity programs enriched with cognitive challenges enhance the effects? A systematic review and meta- analysis', *International Journal of Behavioral Nutrition and Physical Activity*, 4 July 2018. (https://ijbnpa.biomedcentral.com/articles /10.1186/s12966-018-0697-x)
8. 'Heart health declines rapidly after menopause', *American College of Cardiology*, 2 April 2024. (www.acc.org/About-ACC/Press-Releases/ 2024/04/01/21/39/heart-health-declines-rapidly-after-menopause)
9. 'Menopause and your heart', British Heart Foundation. (www.bhf.org. uk/informationsupport/support/women-with-a-heart-condition/ menopause-and-heart-disease)
10. Moilanen, Anna, et al, 'Characteristics of long-term femoral neck bone loss in postmenopausal women: a 25-year follow-up', *Journal of Bone and Mineral Research*, 19 October 2021. (https://onlinelibrary.wiley.com/ doi/10.1002/jbmr.4444)

11. 'Women's Health Strategy needs to go big on osteoporosis emergency affecting one in two women over 50', *Royal Osteoporosis Society*, 30 July 2022. (https://theros.org.uk/latest-news/women-s-health-strategy -needs-to-go-big-on-osteoporosis-emergency-affecting-one-in-two -women-over-50/)
12. Hong, A. Ram and Kim, Sang Wan, 'Effects of resistance exercise on bone health', *Endocrinology and Metabolism*, 30 November 2018. (www.ncbi.nlm.nih.gov/pmc/articles/PMC6279907/)
13. Duggal, Niharika Arora, et al, 'Major features of immunesenescence, including reduced thymic output, are ameliorated by high levels of physical activity in adulthood', *Aging Cell*, 8 March 2018. (www.ncbi. nlm.nih.gov/pmc/articles/PMC5847865/)

CHAPTER 5
1. 'More than one in four sandwich carers report symptoms of mental ill-health', Census, 14 January 2019. (www.ons.gov.uk/people populationandcommunity/healthandsocialcare/healthandwellbeing/ articles/morethanoneinfoursandwichcarersreportsymptomsof mentalillhealth/2019-01-14)
2. 'What is anticipatory grief?', Marie Curie, 1 April 2020. (www. mariecurie.org.uk/talkabout/articles/what-is-anticipatory-grief /271278)
3. 'Key facts and figures about caring', Carers UK. (www.carersuk.org/ policy-and-research/key-facts-and-figures/)
4. 'More than one in four sandwich carers report symptoms of mental ill-health', Census, 14 January 2019. (https://www.ons.gov.uk/ peoplepopulationandcommunity/healthandsocialcare/healthand wellbeing/articles/morethanoneinfoursandwichcarersreport symptomsofmentalillhealth/2019-01-14)
5. Birth characteristics in England and Wales: 2021, Census, 19 January 2023. (www.ons.gov.uk/peoplepopulationandcommunity/birthsdeaths andmarriages/livebirths/bulletins/birthcharacteristicsinengland andwales/2021)
6. 'The divorce gap – women see incomes fall by 33% following divorce, compared to just 18% for men', Legal & General, 4 January 2021. (https://group.legalandgeneral.com/en/newsroom/press-releases/ the-divorce-gap-women-see-incomes-fall-by-33-following-divorce -compared-to-just-18-for-men)

7. Divorce statistics UK 2023, NimbleFins. (www.nimblefins.co.uk/divorce-statistics-uk)

8. 'Young adults living with their parents in low to middle income families', Loughborough University. (www.lboro.ac.uk/research/crsp/our-research/young-adults-living-with-low-middle-income-parents/)

9. 'More adults living with their parents', Office for National Statistics, 10 May 2023. (www.ons.gov.uk/peoplepopulationandcommunity/populationandmigration/populationestimates/articles/moreadultslivingwiththeirparents/2023-05-10)

10. Rozi Jones, 'Income to house price ratio more than doubles since the 70s', *Financial Reporter*, 5 July 2023. (www.financialreporter.co.uk/income-to-house-price-ratio-more-than-doubles-since-the-70s.html)

11. 'Private rental affordability, England, Wales and Northern Ireland: 2022', Census, 23 October 2023. (www.ons.gov.uk/peoplepopulationandcommunity/housing/bulletins/privaterentalaffordabilityengland/2022)

12. Amelia Hill, 'Hidden carers: the sixty-somethings looking after parents and grandchildren', *The Guardian*, 13 February 2017. (www.theguardian.com/membership/2017/feb/13/new-retirement-ageing-responsibility-carers-parents-children-care-crisis)

13. '5 million grandparents take on childcare responsibilities', Age UK, 28 September 2017. (www.ageuk.org.uk/latest-news/articles/2017/september/five-million-grandparents-take-on-childcare-responsibilities/)

CHAPTER 6

1. 'Pelvic floor dysfunction: prevention and non-surgical management', *National Institute for Health and Care Excellence*, 9 December 2021. (www.nice.org.uk/guidance/ng210)

2. 'RCOG calling for action to reduce number of women living with poor pelvic floor health', *Royal College of Obstetricians & Gynaecologists*, 2 February 2023. (www.rcog.org.uk/news/rcog-calling-for-action-to-reduce-number-of-women-living-with-poor-pelvic-floor-health/)

3. Siracusa, Carina and Gray, Amelia, 'Pelvic floor considerations in COVID-19', *Journal of Women's Health Physical Therapy*, 14 October 2020. (www.ncbi.nlm.nih.gov/pmc/articles/PMC7641036/)

4. Milner, Máire, et al, 'Covid-19, pelvic health, and women's voices: a descriptive study', *Continence*, 14 March 2022. (www.ncbi.nlm.nih.gov/pmc/articles/PMC8920089/)

5. 'Bladder and bowel continence care', UK Parliament, 26 June 2023. (https://commonslibrary.parliament.uk/research-briefings/cdp-2023-0145/)

6. Schnelle, John F. and Leung, Felix W., 'Urinary and fecal incontinence in nursing homes', *Gastroenterology*, January 2004. (www.gastrojournal.org/article/S0016-5085(03)01565-8/fulltext)

7. 'RCOG calling for action to reduce number of women living with poor pelvic floor health', *Royal College of Obstetricians & Gynaecologists*, 2 February 2023. (www.rcog.org.uk/news/rcog-calling-for-action-to-reduce-number-of-women-living-with-poor-pelvic-floor-health/)

8. Iglesia, Dr Cheryl, '5 things I wish all women knew about pelvic organ prolapse', *The American College of Obstetricians and Gynecologists*. (www.acog.org/womens-health/experts-and-stories/the-latest/5-things-i-wish-all-women-knew-about-pelvic-organ-prolapse)

CHAPTER 7

1. World Health Organization, Trans fat, 24 January 2024. (www.who.int/news-room/fact-sheets/detail/trans-fat)

2. 'How to get more fibre into your diet', NHS. (www.nhs.uk/live-well/eat-well/digestive-health/how-to-get-more-fibre-into-your-diet/)

3. 'Vitamin D', NHS. (www.nhs.uk/conditions/vitamins-and-minerals/vitamin-d/)

4. Vitamin D testing, NHS. (www.vitamindtest.org.uk/)

5. Dmitrieva, Natalia I., et al, 'Middle-age high normal serum sodium as a risk factor for accelerated biological aging, chronic diseases, and premature mortality', *The Lancet*, Volume 87, January 2023. (www.thelancet.com/journals/ebiom/article/PIIS2352-3964(22)00586-2/fulltext)

6. 'How much water should you drink a day?', BBC, 15 March 2024. (www.bbc.com/future/article/20190403-how-much-water-should-you-drink-a-day)

7. Li, Shizhen, et al, 'Hydration status in older adults: current knowledge and future challenges', 2 June 2023. (www.ncbi.nlm.nih.gov/pmc/articles/PMC10255140/)

8. Mentes, Janet C., et al, 'Salivary osmolality, function, and hydration habits in community-dwelling older adults', *Sage Open Nursing*, 6 February 2019. (https://journals.sagepub.com/doi/full/10.1177/2377960819826253)

9. 'The Eatwell Guide', UK Government, last updated 2 January 2024. (www.gov.uk/government/publications/the-eatwell-guide)

10. Fadnes, Lars T., et al, 'Life expectancy can increase by up to 10 years following sustained shifts towards healthier diets in the United Kingdom', *Nature Food*, 20 November 2023. (www.ncbi.nlm.nih.gov/pmc/articles/PMC10661734/#CR1)

11. Pojednic, Rachele, et al, 'The benefits of physical activity for people with obesity, independent of weight loss: a systematic review', *International Journal of Environmental Research and Public Health*, 20 April 2022. (www.ncbi.nlm.nih.gov/pmc/articles/PMC9102424/)

12. Kodoth, Varna, et al, 'Adverse changes in body composition during the menopausal transition and relation to cardiovascular risk: a contemporary review', *Women's Health Reports*, 13 June 2022. (www.ncbi.nlm.nih.gov/pmc/articles/PMC9258798/)

13. Wu, Yili, et al, 'Sleep duration and obesity among adults: a meta-analysis of prospective studies', *Sleep Medicine*, December 2014. (www.sciencedirect.com/science/article/abs/pii/S1389945714003906?via%3Dihub)

14. Cappuccio, Francesco P., et al, 'Meta-analysis of short sleep duration and obesity in children and adults', *Sleep*, May 2008. (https://pubmed.ncbi.nlm.nih.gov/18517032/)

15. Brown, Stephanie, et al, 'Hypothalamic volume is associated with body mass index', *NeuroImage: Clinical*, 2023. (www.sciencedirect.com/science/article/pii/S2213158223001699?via%3Dihub)

16. Campbell, Bill, et al, 'International Society of Sports Nutrition position stand: protein and exercise', *Journal of the International Society of Sports Nutrition*, 26 September 2007. (www.ncbi.nlm.nih.gov/pmc/articles/PMC2117006/)

17. Kessler, Katharina and Pivovarova-Ramich, Olga, 'Meal timing, aging, and metabolic health', *International Journal of Molecular Sciences*, 18 April 2019. (www.ncbi.nlm.nih.gov/pmc/articles/PMC6514931/)

18. Dr Lisa Mosconi, *The Menopause Brain* (Atlantic Books, 2024), p.208

19. 'The disconnected mind', Age UK. (www.ageuk.org.uk/our-impact/policy-research/what-we-research/the-disconnected-mind/)

20. Kirwan, Richard P., et al, 'Protein interventions augment the effect of resistance exercise on appendicular lean mass and handgrip strength in older adults: a systematic review and meta-analysis of randomized controlled trials', *American Journal of Clinical Nutrition*, 4 March 2022. (https://pubmed.ncbi.nlm.nih.gov/34673936/)

21. Morris, Susan, et al, 'Inadequacy of protein intake in older UK adults', *Geriatrics*, 2020. (www.mdpi.com/2308-3417/5/1/6)

22. Merriam Webster Dictionary. (www.merriam-webster.com/dictionary/diet)

23. Gerber, Mariette and Hoffman, Richard, 'The Mediterranean diet: health, science and society', *British Journal of Nutrition*, April 2015. (https://pubmed.ncbi.nlm.nih.gov/26148921/)

24. Tor-Roca, Alba, et al, 'A Mediterranean Diet-based metabolomic score and cognitive decline in older adults: a case–control analysis nested within the three-city cohort study', *Molecular Nutrition & Food Research*, 24 October 2023. (https://onlinelibrary.wiley.com/doi/10.1002/mnfr.202300271)

25. Mazza, Elisa, et al, 'Mediterranean Diet in healthy aging', *Journal of Nutritional Health & Aging*, 15 September 2021. (www.ncbi.nlm.nih.gov/pmc/articles/PMC8442641/)

26. Hinzey, Elaine and Chien, Shanley, 'Mediterranean Diet: beginner's guide to a healthy heart', *US News and World Report*, 14 May 2024. (https://health.usnews.com/best-diet/mediterranean-diet)

27. Buettner, Dan and Skemp, Sam, 'Blue Zones', *American Journal of Lifestyle Medicine*, 17 July 2016. (www.ncbi.nlm.nih.gov/pmc/articles/PMC6125071/)

28. Buettner, Dan, 'The World's 6th Blue Zones Region – an engineered longevity hotspot'. (www.bluezones.com/2023/10/the-worlds-6th-blue-zones-region/#)

29. https://www.nih.gov/

30. Hypertension, World Health Organization, 16 March 2023. (www.who.int/news-room/fact-sheets/detail/hypertension)

31. Health Survey for England, 2021 part 2, NHS. (https://digital.nhs.uk/data-and-information/publications/statistical/health-survey-for-england/2021-part-2/adult-health-hypertension)

32. 'Risk factors for undiagnosed high blood pressure in England: 2015 to 2019', Office for National Statistics, 27 April 2023. (www.ons.gov.uk/peoplepopulationandcommunity/healthandsocialcare/healthand

wellbeing/articles/riskfactorsforundiagnosedhighbloodpressurein england/2015to2019)

33. British and Irish Hypertension Society. (https://bihsoc.org/bp -monitors/for-home-use/)

34. Challa, Hima J., et al, 'DASH diet to stop hypertension', *StatPearls* 23 January 2023. (www.ncbi.nlm.nih.gov/books/NBK482514/)

35. Onwuzo, Chidera, et al, 'DASH diet: a review of its scientifically proven hypertension reduction and health benefits', *Cureus*, 4 September 2023. (www.ncbi.nlm.nih.gov/pmc/articles/PMC10551663/)

36. Morris, Martha Clare, et al, 'MIND diet slows cognitive decline with aging', *Alzheimers & Dementia*, September 2015. (www.ncbi.nlm.nih.gov/pmc/articles/PMC4581900/)

37. Ibid

38. Kheirouri, Sorayya and Alizadeh, Mohammad , 'MIND diet and cognitive performance in older adults: a systematic review', *Critical Reviews in Food Science & Nutrition*, 14 May 2021. (https://pubmed.ncbi.nlm.nih.gov/33989093/)

39. Tangney, Christy C, et al, 'Relation of DASH- and Mediterranean-like dietary patterns to cognitive decline in older persons', *Neurology*, 14 October 2014. (www.ncbi.nlm.nih.gov/pmc/articles/PMC4206157/)

40. Health Survey for England, 2022, part 1, NHS, 6 June 2024. (https://digital.nhs.uk/data-and-information/publications/statistical/health -survey-for-england/2022-part-1)

41. Peschke, Elmar and Mühlbauer, Eckhard, 'New evidence for a role of melatonin in glucose regulation', *Best Practice & Research Clinical Endocrinology & Metabolism*, October 2010. (www.sciencedirect.com/science/article/abs/pii/S1521690X10001168)

42. Bonilla, Diego A., et al, 'The 4R's Framework of Nutritional Strategies for Post-Exercise Recovery: A Review with Emphasis on New Generation of Carbohydrates', *International Journal of Environmental Research and Public Health*, 25 December 2020. (www.ncbi.nlm.nih.gov/pmc/articles/PMC7796021/)

43. Nutrasource (https://certifications.nutrasource.ca/certified-products ?type=certification&value=IFOS)

44. Liao, Chun-De, et al, 'Comparative efficacy of different protein supplements on muscle mass, strength, and physical indices of sarcopenia among community-dwelling, hospitalized or

institutionalized older adults undergoing resistance training: a
network meta-analysis of randomized controlled trials', *Nutrients*,
25 March 2024. (www.mdpi.com/2072-6643/16/7/941)

45. Kreider, Richard B., et al, 'International Society of Sports Nutrition
position stand: safety and efficacy of creatine supplementation in
exercise, sport, and medicine', *Journal of the International Society of
Sports Nutrition*, 13 June 2017. (https://jissn.biomedcentral.com/articles/
10.1186/s12970-017-0173-z)

46. Smith-Ryan, Abbie E., et al, 'Creatine supplementation in women's
health: a lifespan perspective', *Nutrients*, 15 January 2021. (www.mdpi.
com/2072-6643/13/3/877)

47. Ellery, Stacey, et al, 'Creatine for women: a review of the relationship
between creatine and the reproductive cycle and female-specific
benefits of creatine therapy', *Amino Acids*, August 2016. (www.
researchgate.net/publication/295540299_Creatine_for_women_a_
review_of_the_relationship_between_creatine_and_the_reproductive_
cycle_and_female-specific_benefits_of_creatine_therapy)

CHAPTER 8

1. Borg, Gunnar A.V., 'Psychophysical bases of perceived exertion',
Medicine & Science in Sports & Exercise, 1982. (https://journals.lww.com/
acsm-msse/abstract/1982/05000/psychophysical_bases_of_perceived
_exertion.12.aspx)

CHAPTER 12

1. Lu, Chang-bo, et al, 'Musculoskeletal pain during the menopausal
transition: a systematic review and meta-analysis', *Neural Plasticity*, 25
November 2020. (www.ncbi.nlm.nih.gov/pmc/articles/PMC7710408/)

2. Wright, Vonda J., et al, 'The musculoskeletal syndrome of menopause',
Climateric, 30 July 2024. (https://doi.org/10.1080/13697137.2024.
2380363)

3. Monteagudo, Manuel, et al, 'Plantar fasciopathy', *EFORT Open Review*,
29 August 2018. (www.ncbi.nlm.nih.gov/pmc/articles/PMC6134886/)

4. Rathleff, Michael, 'Plantar fasciitis – important new research by
Michael Rathleff', *British Journal of Sports Medicine*, 15 September 2014.
(https://blogs.bmj.com/bjsm/2014/09/15/plantar-fasciitis-important
-new-research-by-michael-rathleff/)

5. Jibri, Zaid, et al, 'Patellar maltracking: an update on the diagnosis and treatment strategies', *Insights into Imaging*, 14 June 2019. (www.ncbi. nlm.nih.gov/pmc/articles/PMC6570735/)

6. Harvey, D., 'Assessment of the flexibility of elite athletes using the modified Thomas Test', *British Journal of Sports Medicine*, 1998. (www. ncbi.nlm.nih.gov/pmc/articles/PMC1756061/pdf/v032p00068.pdf)

7. 'Hormone therapy appears to reduce risk of shoulder pain in older women', *Duke Health*, 11 October 2022. (https://corporate.dukehealth. org/news/hormone-therapy-appears-reduce-risk-shoulder-pain -older-women)

CHAPTER 13

1. Blume, Christine, et al, 'Effects of light on human circadian rhythms, sleep and mood', *Somnologie*, 20 August 2019. (www.ncbi.nlm.nih.gov /pmc/articles/PMC6751071/)